RAND

Analysis of the Children's Hospital Graduate Medical Education Program Fund Allocations for Indirect Medical Education Costs

Barbara O. Wynn, Jennifer Kawata

Prepared for the
Health Resources and Services Administration

RAND Health

The research described in this report was sponsored by the Health Resources and Services Administration. The research was conducted within RAND Health.

ISBN: 0-8330-3183-X

RAND is a nonprofit institution that helps improve policy and decisionmaking through research and analysis. RAND® is a registered trademark. RAND's publications do not necessarily reflect the opinions or policies of its research sponsors.

Published 2002 by RAND
1700 Main Street, P.O. Box 2138, Santa Monica, CA 90407-2138
1200 South Hayes Street, Arlington, VA 22202-5050
201 North Craig Street, Suite 102, Pittsburgh, PA 15213
RAND URL: http://www.rand.org/
To order RAND documents or to obtain additional information, contact Distribution Services: Telephone: (310) 451-7002; Fax: (310) 451-6915; Email: order@rand.org

PREFACE

In FY2000, the Public Health Service Act was amended to establish a Children's Hospital Graduate Medical Education (CHGME) program to support graduate medical education in children's hospitals. The Health Resources and Services Administration (HRSA) in the Department of Health and Human Services administers the program.

The CHGME program provides funding for both the direct and indirect medical education costs associated with operating approved GME programs. Funding for the indirect medical education costs is based on the indirect expenses associated with the treatment of more severely ill patients and the additional patient care costs related to residency training programs. HRSA elected to use the current Medicare formula for hospital inpatient operating costs to establish the initial amounts allocated to each eligible children's teaching hospital for indirect medical education costs. A hospital's allocation is a function of its discharges, case mix index, ratio of residents-to-beds and the average hourly wages in the geographic area in which the hospital is located.

HRSA asked RAND to undertake a number of activities related to implementation of the CHGME program. This HRSA-sponsored study reports on our analysis of issues related to estimating indirect medical education costs specific to pediatric discharges. It uses multivariate regression analysis to investigate the effect of residency training programs on pediatric costs per discharge using different measures of teaching intensity, including residents-to-beds and residents-to-average daily census. The study uses the coefficients from regressions to establish potential allocation formulae for indirect medical education funds that could be used by the CHGME program in lieu of the Medicare formula.

CONTENTS

TABLES AND FIGURES

SUMMARY

PURPOSE

Public Law No. 106-129 amended the Public Health Service Act to establish a new Children's Hospital Graduate Medical Education (CHGME) program to support graduate medical education (GME) in children's hospitals. The provision authorizes payments for both the direct (DGME) and indirect medical education (IME) costs associated with operating approved GME programs.

With respect to the IME funds, the statute requires the Secretary to determine an amount based on the indirect expenses associated with the treatment of more severely ill patients and the additional patient care costs related to residency training programs. The Health Resources and Services Administration (HRSA) has elected to use the current Medicare formula for hospital inpatient operating costs to establish the IME allocation factor for the CHGME program. A hospital's allocation is a function of its discharges, case mix index, ratio of residents-to-beds and the average hourly wages in the geographic area in which the hospital is located. A hospital's IME factor increases 6.5 percent for each .10 increment in its ratio of residents-to-beds.

This report explores issues related to estimating IME costs specific to pediatric discharges. It uses multivariate regression analysis to investigate the effect of residency training programs on pediatric costs per discharge using different measures of teaching intensity, including residents-to-beds and residents-to-average daily census. The study uses the coefficients from regressions to establish potential IME allocation formulae that could be used by the CHGME program and to estimate the aggregate IME costs of children's teaching hospitals.

ORGANIZATION OF REPORT AND SUMMARY OF FINDINGS

Section 1 of this report provides an overview of the CHGME provisions related to IME funds. It establishes a policy framework for viewing IME funding as a mechanism for "leveling the playing field" for children's teaching hospitals so that they can compete more effectively with other hospitals for pediatric patients. The Medicare program's IME adjustments to its prospective payments for inpatient hospital services can be used as prototypes for determining potential IME allocation factors for the CHGME program. The IME effect on a hospital's average cost per pediatric discharge can be determined through multivariate regression analysis. The regressions can be "fully-specified" (i.e., include a full set of independent variables that explain the variation in average costs for pediatric discharges across hospitals) or they can be "payer" regressions that include a more limited set of independent variables. A payer regression includes as independent variables only those factors that third-party payers are likely to recognize in purchasing pediatric inpatient care, such as case mix and geographic differences in wage levels. Key policy issues that need to be addressed in performing the multivariate analyses are:

- Whether the dependent variable should be the average cost per pediatric stay in all community hospitals or only in children's hospitals; and,
- Which factors in addition to a teaching intensity measure should be included as independent variables.

Section 2 provides information on the data sources and methods we use to examine potential IME allocation factors. We draw on data from several sources to develop our analysis file. The most important sources are 100% claims data from 11 states participating in the Hospital Cost and Utilization Project and Medicare cost reports for these hospitals. The states are: Arizona, California, Colorado, Florida, Iowa, Maryland, Massachusetts, New York, Oregon, Washington, and Wisconsin. They account for about 36 percent of total pediatric discharges and include several states with children's teaching hospitals. We link the claims data and cost report data for the hospitals in our analysis file and combine the data in several ways:

- For each hospital in the analysis file, we estimate the cost for each pediatric discharge, its average cost per pediatric discharge by HCFA DRG, and its average cost for all pediatric discharges.

- We construct a set of DRG relative weights based on the costs of pediatric discharges in our analysis file. We use Medicare payment parameters for the hospital wage index, IME and serving low-income patients to standardize each hospital's costs for factors that have a systematic effect on costs per discharge. A DRG's relative weight is based on the ratio of the average standardized cost per pediatric discharge in that DRG across all hospitals to the average standardized cost for all pediatric discharges across all hospitals.

- We construct two case mix indices for each hospital: a HCFA CMI based on the HCFA version 16 relative weights (derived from Medicare costs per discharge) and a "Pediatric CMI" based on the relative weights derived from the standardized costs for pediatric discharges.

Our primary analysis tool in investigating IME costs per discharge for pediatric patients is multivariate regressions using each hospital's average cost per pediatric discharge as the dependent variable. We investigate the impact of using different measures of teaching intensity and case mix as independent variables. The teaching intensity measures include the two utilized by the Medicare program (ratio of residents-to beds and ratio of residents-to-average daily census) as well as two measures that provide greater weight to outpatient care. The latter are the number of full-time equivalent (FTE) residents and the ratio of residents to an average daily census adjusted for outpatient services. We also examine the impact that the inclusion or exclusion of other variables has on the teaching intensity coefficient. In this regard, we focus in the payer regressions on factors that are treated differently by HCFA and the Medicare Payment Advisory Commission (MedPAC) in estimating the Medicare IME adjustment. These variables account for the hospital's volume of "outlier" or high cost cases and its proportion of low-income patients.

We use the coefficients from the payer regressions to establish potential IME allocation factors. Using these factors and available information on children's teaching hospitals, we model how IME funds would be allocated by the CHGME using the IME allocation factors derived from the regressions and compare the results to the allocations using the Medicare formulae. Our ability to model the effects of potential allocation factors is limited by available data for children's teaching hospitals to those using HCFA v.16 relative weights. We also use the regression coefficients to estimate aggregate IME costs for children's teaching hospitals.

We present our results in Section 3. Key findings include the following:

- In fully specified regressions that include a full set of explanatory variables, the teaching variable is a significant factor in explaining differences in costs per discharge for pediatric patients. In discharge-weighted regressions, cost per discharge increases 2.1 percent for each .10 increment in the ratio of residents-to-average daily census.

- The inclusion or exclusion of other explanatory variables affects the size of the teaching coefficient. In particular, the variable for outlier cases (defined as atypical cases with long lengths of stay) has a strong influence on the teaching coefficient. When outlier cases are included in a payer regression, cost per case increases 4.13 percent for each .10 increment in the residents-to-average daily census ratio. When outlier cases are excluded, cost per case increases 7.47 percent for each .10 increment in the ratio.

- The regression results indicate that improvements in the case mix index would improve the teaching estimates. When the pediatric CMI is substituted for the HCFA CMI in the fully specified regressions, the significance of CMI increases while the coefficients for both the teaching and outlier variables decrease significantly.

- The choices between using residents-to-beds or residents-to-average daily census as the measure of teaching intensity and between using different forms of these measures (e.g., logged or non-logged) do not produce marked differences in the size of the teaching estimate. The teaching effect on cost per discharge is lower when the number of residents is used as the teaching measure and higher when the ratio of residents-to-average daily census is adjusted for outpatient volume.

- The choice of teaching measure affects the distribution of IME funds across children's teaching hospitals. Using the Medicare formula as the baseline, the largest redistribution occurs when the allocations are based on the number of residents only. Whether these redistributions would be appropriate depends on the policy objectives for the CHGME fund.

- The estimate of total IME costs at children's teaching hospitals for inpatient services only is dependent on the other factors included in the estimate. For inpatient services only, total IME costs are an estimated $830 million using either residents-to-average daily census or residents-to-beds as the teaching measure and controlling for case mix and geographic wage differences only. This compares to $620 million using the Medicare payment parameters. The higher teaching estimate may result from the shortcomings in the ability of the HCFA DRGs and relative weights to account for severity differences in pediatric inpatient stays.

We discuss the major findings and our conclusions in Section 4. We believe the study results indicate that the Medicare IME formula is a reasonable basis for allocating IME funds under the CHGME program. For the most part, the allocations are similar to those based on pediatric costs per case using either residents-to-beds or residents-to-average daily census as the teaching measure. Nevertheless, there are aspects of the methodology that warrant further investigation. In particular, refinements in case mix measurement could improve the estimates of IME costs and how the IME funds are allocated across children's teaching hospitals. Data became available as this study was nearing completion that would permit an analysis of whether more refined DRG classification systems such as APR-DRGs would have a significant impact on the allocation of IME funds. This data could also be used to examine the issue of how including an outlier variable would affect the allocations.

Another area that warrants additional attention concerns outpatient services. The simulation results indicate that switching to a teaching measure that takes outpatient volume into account could involve significant redistributions for some children's teaching hospitals. The adjustment that we investigated for outpatient volume assumes the IME effect on outpatient services is comparable to the effect on inpatient services. This is an empirical question that would benefit from further analysis. However, the lack of consistent measures of outpatient volume and case mix will make it difficult to explore this issue.

ACKNOWLEDGMENTS

We are grateful for the valuable support that we received throughout this study from our HRSA Project Officer, Emily DeCoster. We also appreciate the time and energy that several other HRSA officials devoted to the project. In particular, we are extremely grateful for the insightful comments provided by Dr. Ayah Johnson on an earlier version of this report and for the support provided by Dr. Lawrence Clare and Dr. Barbara Brookmyer at the start of the project. We also appreciate the assistance provided by Stephen Phillips and Miechal Lefkowitz of the Health Care Financing Administration in providing data needed for our analyses. Finally, we appreciate the thoughtful comments of Jeffrey Wasserman, Ph.D. and Jeannette Rogowski, Ph.D., of RAND in reviewing this report.

GLOSSARY, LIST OF SYMBOLS, ETC.

Symbol	Definition
ADC	Average daily census
AHRQ	Agency for Healthcare Research and Quality
AP-DRGs	All Payer Diagnosis- related Groups
APR-DRG	All Payer Refined Diagnosis- related Groups
CHGME	Children's Hospital Graduate Medical School
CMI	Case mix index
DGME	Direct graduate medical education
GME	Graduate medical education
DRG	Diagnosis- related Group
HCFA	Health Care Financing Administration (now Centers for Medicare and Medicaid Services)
HCUP	Hospital Cost and Utilization Project
HRSA	Health Resources and Services Administration
IME	Indirect medical education
MDC	Major Diagnostic Catagory
MedPAC	Medicare Payment Advisory Commission
NACHRI	National Association of Children's Hospitals and Related Institutions
NOD	Number of Discharges
PPS	Prospective payment system
TI	Teaching intensity
UHDDS	Uniform Hospital Discharge Data Set
WF	Weighting Factor
WI	Wage index

1. OVERVIEW OF INDIRECT MEDICAL EDUCATION FUNDING

The legislation authorizing the CHGME fund provides for an IME payment based on the indirect expenses associated with the treatment of more severely ill patients and the additional costs related to residency training programs. In determining the appropriate payment amount, the Secretary is to take into account:

- The variation in case mix among children's hospitals; and,
- The number of full-time equivalent (FTE) residents in approved training programs at each eligible children's teaching hospital.

The initial legislation authorized the following amounts for the CHGME fund:

- IME: $190 million in FY2000 and again in FY2001
- DGME: $90 million in FY 2000 and $95 million in FY2001

The total FY2000 appropriation for both DGME and IME was $40 million, considerably less than the authorized amounts. HRSA allocated 2/3 of this amount for IME funding and used the Medicare IME formula for hospital operating costs to establish each children's hospital's share of the IME funds. In FY2001, the total appropriation for the CHGME fund increased to $235 million. HRSA used the same methodology with minor modifications to allocate the FY2001 funds (DHHS, 2001b).

In the subsections that follow, we discuss the conceptual framework for funding IME costs in children's teaching hospitals, review case mix measurement systems that could be used to account for differences in the types of patients treated by children's teaching hospitals, and highlight policy issues that should be considered in allocating IME funds to children's teaching hospitals.

CONCEPTUAL FRAMEWORK FOR FUNDING IME COSTS

The IME funds compensate eligible children's hospitals for higher indirect expenses associated with residency training programs. The IME costs are systematically higher costs associated with teaching activity that cannot be accounted for by other factors, including patient severity that is not measured by the patient classification system and case mix index (i.e., within DRG severity).[1] These higher costs are generally associated with treating a patient population with more complex needs than non-teaching hospitals and with more resource-intensive treatment patterns when residents are involved in the care of patients (e.g., more diagnostic tests) (Anderson and Lave, 1986; Thorpe, 1988; Sheingold, 1990; Dalton, Norton and Kilpatrick, 2001; COGME, 2001). Since teaching hospitals tend to have higher costs per case relative to other hospitals in the same area with comparable case mix, they may not be able to compete successfully for patients if they need to price their services to cover the higher costs associated with the teaching program (Commonwealth, 1997; Mechanic, Coleman and Dobson, 1998; COGME, 2001). In contrast to general community hospitals, children's teaching hospitals receive little or no support from Medicare for graduate medical education. Paying for the indirect expenses for teaching activities through the CHGME fund "levels the playing field" and allows children's teaching hospitals to price their services more competitively (DHHS, 2001a).

For the CHGME fund, the basic policy questions are: 1) the level of funding that should be provided for IME costs through the CHGME program and 2) how the IME funds should be distributed among the children's teaching hospitals. Multivariate regression analyses that examine the relationship between teaching intensity and other factors on patient care costs can inform both policy questions. With regard to the first question, the regression results can be used to estimate aggregate IME costs across children's teaching hospitals and to support the decision regarding how available CHME funds are divided between DGME and IME support. Full funding of IME costs through the CHGME program is not needed to "level the playing field." To differing degrees, children's teaching hospitals are able to compete on quality as well as price and they receive support for IME costs through other sources, such as the

---

[1] As explained in greater detail below, a patient classification system (e.g., diagnosis-related groups) is used to measure the resource intensity of stays across classes of patients and to compare the mix of patients treated by different hospitals. The case mix index measures the hospital's average resource intensity for inpatient stays.

Medicaid program and other payers, philanthropy and endowment funds. Thus, the determination of the appropriate level of support rests on policy considerations informed by empirical analyses. This study is limited to estimating total IME costs for children's teaching hospitals and does not address directly the question of the appropriate level of support.

With regard to the allocation of IME funds, the regression results that are used to estimate total IME costs can also be used to develop potential formulae for allocating IME funds among eligible children's teaching hospitals. However, the results are highly dependent on how the regressions are specified and the choice among technically correct specifications rests on policy considerations. These considerations include the precedence of the Medicare program, an assessment of which cost factors should be supported through IME funding, and whether to include outpatient services in the allocation formula.

MEDICARE IME ADJUSTMENT

Medicare's prospective payment system for hospital inpatient services has separate standard payment rates for operating and capital-related costs. An adjustment is made to the standard payment rates for the indirect costs associated with teaching activities. [2] The adjustments for operating costs and capital-related costs are different:

- The IME adjustment to the standard payment for operating costs is established by statute and exceeds an analytically justified level. The current adjustment formula increases payment approximately 6.5 percent for each .10-point increase in the ratio of residents-to-beds.[3] This formula is also used by the Department of Defense to adjust TRICARE payments

---

[2] The standard payment rates are the wage-adjusted DRG payment rates before adjustment for IME, for serving a disproportionate share of low-income patients (DSH), and high-cost outlier cases.

[3] The original estimate was 4.05 and was doubled when PPS was implemented. Over time, the factor has been reduced from 2.0 $(1+\text{resident-to-bed ratio}^{.405} -1)$ to 1.86 $(1+\text{resident-to-bed ratio}^{.405} -1)$, or 6.5 percent. Under the Benefits Improvement and Protection Act of 2000 (P.L. 106-554), the multiplier will be reduced to 1.35 in FY2003 and thereafter, resulting in a 5.5 percent adjustment.

to children's teaching hospitals following its general use of Medicare facility-level payment parameters.

- The IME adjustment to the prospective payment for capital-related costs was established administratively in FY1992 based an analysis of the effect of teaching on total (operating and capital) costs per case (HCFA, 1991). The adjustment formula increases payment approximately 2.8 percentage points for every .10 increment in the hospital's ratio of residents-to-average daily census (i.e., the average number of inpatients per day in the hospital).

The Medicare Payment Advisory Commission (MedPAC) recently re-estimated the indirect teaching effect on total inpatient costs per case at 3.1 percent for each .10-point increment in the ratio of residents-to-beds.[4] Medicare does not make an IME adjustment in its payments to teaching hospitals for outpatient services because HCFA found the teaching effect on outpatient facility costs was small (DHHS, 1998).

DETERMINING THE IME FORMULA

Traditionally, the indirect expenses associated with teaching activity are estimated through multivariate regression analysis. For inpatient hospital services, the dependent variable is cost per discharge (exclusive of DGME costs) at a particular hospital and the independent variables are factors that explain costs, such as the case mix and the wage index. The general specification is that:

C   = f (CMI, WI, X), where:

C   = average cost per case at the facility

CMI   = the case mix index for the facility

WI   = the wage index for the geographic area, and

X   = a vector of additional explanatory variables that affect a hospital's costs per case, such as its teaching activities, proportion of low-income patients, number of beds, etc.

---

[4]Personal communication with Craig Lisk, MedPAC staff. The Commission's estimate for operating costs only is 3.2 percent per 10 percentage point increment in teaching intensity (MedPAC, 2000).

"Fully specified" regressions include a number of independent variables that explain the variation in average cost per discharge across hospitals. These include variables related to the hospital's geographic location, its size and infrastructure, and the characteristics of its patient population. These regressions are used to understand the factors that have an effect on costs per discharge. "Payer" regressions include a more limited set of independent variables, namely, those factors that are likely to be recognized by third-party payers in purchasing hospital care. Payer regression models have been used to estimate the Medicare IME adjustment. While some regression equations may provide a better fit than others, there is no single "correct" specification. The choice of variables in a payer regression involves policy considerations that affect the IME estimate. For example, HCFA's IME estimate that is used in the Medicare capital prospective payment system includes case mix, the hospital wage index, teaching intensity, low-income patient population, and large urban location as independent variables (DHHS, 1991). The MedPAC regression includes a variable for atypically high cost or "outlier" cases but does not include a low-income patient variable. The different specifications are based on policy differences regarding which factors should be controlled for in determining the IME adjustment (and not paid for as part of the IME adjustment) and which factors should be recognized through the IME adjustment.

The coefficients from the regression results can be used to establish empirically justified factors for the independent variables, including an IME factor for the CHGME fund. However, studies have shown that the coefficients are highly dependent on the variables included in the model and the way the equation is specified (Anderson and Lave, 1986; Thorpe, 1988; Sheingold, 1990; Mechanic et al, 1998). Teaching intensity is positively correlated with a number of the other variables, including size, proportion of outlier cases and percentage of low-income patients. The exclusion of these variables "loads" some of their effect onto the teaching coefficient. The underlying policy issue is the extent to which these other factors affecting cost per case should be supported by IME payments.

CASE MIX MEASUREMENT

Case mix refers to the mix of patients treated by the hospital. A patient classification system is used to measure the relative resource intensity of stays across classes of patients and to compare the mix of patients treated by different hospitals.

PATIENT CLASSIFICATION SYSTEMS

There are case mix classification systems that use information available on the Uniform Hospital Discharge Data Set (UHDDS) to group patients that have similar clinical characteristics and require similar levels of resources. The information includes: principal and secondary diagnoses, complications and co-morbidities, surgical procedures, age, sex and discharge destination.[5] Below we briefly discuss four systems used to classify patients into diagnosis-related groups (DRGs) using UHDDS information.

HCFA DRGs. The HCFA DRGs are used by the Medicare program and have been adopted by Medicaid in some States. Since the original DRGs were implemented in FY1984, HCFA's DRG classification refinement activity has concentrated on the Medicare population and has not incorporated significant refinements in the pediatric and neonate classifications. The relative weights are derived from Medicare claims data and are not as suitable for making case-mix comparisons for pediatric cases as other systems. The principal advantage to using the HCFA DRGs is that they are widely used and the grouping logic is in the public domain. In particular, the Agency for Healthcare Research and Quality uses the HCFA DRGs in partnership with 22 States in the Hospital Cost and Utilization Project (HCUP). HCUP consists of two databases. The state inpatient databases (SID) contain 100% of the claims data for each of the 22

---

[5]Birthweight, which is not a UHDDS data element, is used in some systems to classify neonates and can be developed from the fifth digit of the ICD-9-CM prematurity diagnosis codes. For detailed comparisons of the differences in the grouping logic and performance of these systems in explaining cost variations see: Norbert Goldfield, M.D., Editor, Physician Profiling and Risk Adjustment, 2nd Edition, Aspen Publishers, 1999 and John H. Muldoon, "Structure and Performance of Different DRG Classification Systems for Neonatal Medicine," Supplement of Evidence-Based Quality Improvement in Neonatal and Perinatal Medicine, Pediatrics, Vol. 103, No.1 January 1, 1999.

participating states. The nationwide inpatient sample (NIS) includes 100% of the claims data from a 20% sample of the hospitals in the 22 States.

All Payer DRGs. The All-Payer (AP) DRGs were developed by 3M HIS for the New York State Department of Health. The AP-DRGs include refinements to the neonate and pediatric DRGs developed by the National Association of Children's Hospitals and Related Institutions (NACHRI). HCFA DRGs have seven groups for neonates; in contrast, the AP-DRGs have 34 groupings that include six birth weight ranges as a grouping variable along with breakouts for surgical and medical cases. In addition, the AP-DRGs establish groupings for major complications and co-morbidities that have greater impact on hospital resource use than the principal diagnosis. The AP-DRG system is a proprietary system that requires a licensing fee to use.

TRICARE/CHAMPUS DRGs. The prospective payment system used by the Department of Defense (DoD) to pay civilian providers is modeled on the Medicare prospective payment system. (Unlike Medicare, however, children's hospitals are included.) DoD uses the HCFA DRG classification system with several modifications for pediatric cases, including adopting the 34 neo-natal DRGs used by the AP-DRGs in place of the HCFA DRGs for neonates. Also, the TRICARE/CHAMPUS relative weights are based on claims for the TRICARE population.

All Payer Refined DRGs. Building on the base AP-DRGs (prior to subdividing for complications and co-morbidities), the All Payer Refined (APR-) DRGs assign three descriptors to each patient: the base APR-DRG, a severity of illness subgroup, and a risk of mortality subgroup. Principal diagnosis and surgical procedures determine the base APR-DRG. There are four severity of illness and four risk of mortality subgroups. The subgroups take into account the interaction between the principal and secondary diagnoses, age, and certain non-operating room procedures. Assignment is specific for each base AP-DRG. For evaluating resource use, the APR-DRGs in conjunction with the severity of illness subgroups is used. The APR-DRGs are a proprietary system that was jointly developed by 3M HIS and NACHRI.

A comparative study by 3M HIS and NACHRI using 1993 sample claims data evaluated how well various DRG systems predicted cost at the hospital level (Averill et al., 1999). A 20 percent sample of claims for 40 children's hospitals was included in the analysis. Overall, the study found that APR-DRGs are a better predictor of resource use for inpatient stays at children's hospitals. However, most improvement over the HCFA DRGs and AP-DRGs was in neonate cases, which were 8 percent of the cases in the children's hospital sample (TRICARE/CHAMPUS DRGs were not separately evaluated). Since IME funds are allocated at the facility-level, differences in the patient classification system are important only if they capture systematic differences in the types of patients treated at various classes of children's teaching hospitals. The poorer performance of the HCFA DRGs in predicting the costs of neonates is problematic if there are systematic differences in the types of neonates treated at various children's teaching hospitals. We do not have patient-level data from children's teaching hospitals that would allow us to investigate this question as part of this study.

DRG RELATIVE WEIGHTS AND CASE MIX INDEX

Each DRG is assigned a relative weight based on the average resources required to treat patients in the DRG relative to the average discharge. A hospital's case mix index is the average DRG relative weight for its inpatients, i.e., the sum of the DRG relative weights for inpatient stays in the hospital divided by the total number of inpatient stays. Thus, the patient population used to derive the relative weights is an important factor in determining the hospital's case mix index. Medicare uses relative weights derived from billing data for Medicare patients. Individuals entitled to Medicare benefits include those who are over age 65, are disabled, or have end-stage renal disease. Some DRGs are specific to patients age 0-17. Since Medicare has relatively few pediatric cases, FY1996 relative weights for these DRGs were supplemented by data from 19 states. Since that time, the relative weights for the low-volume DRGs (those with less than 10 Medicare cases) have not been updated for changes in practice patterns. Other DRGs to which pediatric cases may be assigned are applicable to all age groups.

The relative weights for these DRGs are recalibrated annually based on Medicare data for a predominately aged population. Some states have developed relative weights specific to their Medicaid population while others use relative weights based on a national sample of all patients. The APR-DRG relative weights developed by NACHRI/3M HIS are based on a national sample of acute general hospitals and most children's hospitals.

In the FY2000 grants process for CHGME, HRSA elected to use the HCFA DRG Version 15 (classification system and relative weights) in the IME allocation formula. Differences in the DRG relative weights attributable to using Medicare discharge data instead of pediatric discharge data are important only if they affect the allocation of IME funds to individual children's teaching hospitals. We do not have patient-level data for children's teaching hospitals that would allow us to investigate this issue as part of this study.

CONSIDERATIONS FOR THE CHGME FUND

The Medicare estimates of the IME effect on teaching hospital costs are based on Medicare costs per discharge and case mix information. The estimates serve as a prototype for determining an IME allocation factor for children's teaching hospitals. However, we do not know 1) if teaching has a similar effect on costs for pediatric inpatients as it does for Medicare patients, 2) if there are systematic case mix differences across children's teaching hospitals that are not measured by the HCFA DRGs and relative weights, and 3) how the costs of pediatric care in children's teaching hospitals compare to the costs in other hospitals.

In this report, we begin to address the first two questions. We estimate the effect of teaching activity on pediatric costs per case and the sensitivity of those estimates to using case mix indices derived from pediatric data relative to Medicare data. We also explore the sensitivity of the CHGME fund distributions to different measures of teaching intensity. We highlight below the major considerations for establishing the IME allocation factor. These considerations form the framework for our analyses and include the following issues:

- What is the basic purpose of the IME funding? Is it to recognize a) the higher costs of treating children in teaching hospitals (both general and children's) relative to non-teaching hospitals, b) the higher costs of children's teaching hospitals relative to children's hospitals that are not engaged in teaching, or c) the higher costs of children's teaching hospitals relative to all other hospitals?

- What are the implications of using more refined measures of case mix in children's teaching hospitals?

- To what extent should other factors affecting costs (e.g., serving low-income patients) be supported by IME funding?

- How should teaching intensity be measured? Should it draw on the Medicare program (using either residents-to-beds or residents-to-average daily census) or should it include outpatient services?

Purpose of the Adjustment

A key issue in estimating the IME effect is which hospitals should be included in the analysis. The underlying policy question is whether the adjustment is to recognize a) the higher costs of treating children in teaching hospitals (both general and children's) relative to non-teaching hospitals, b) the higher costs of children's teaching hospitals relative to children's hospitals that are not engaged in teaching, or c) the higher costs of children's teaching hospitals relative to all other hospitals? The answer will determine which hospitals are included in an estimate of IME costs. Assuming that the adjustment is intended to "level the playing field," using all facilities with pediatric cases to estimate the IME effect on costs is more appropriate than confining the analysis to children's hospitals. With the exception of a few markets such as Philadelphia, children's hospitals do not share the same market area. Support is needed for the IME costs they incur relative to other hospitals that provide care to pediatric patients in their market. Accordingly, we base our IME estimate on costs incurred by a broadly representative group of hospitals in providing care to pediatric patients.

Ideally, we would include children's hospitals in the analysis so that we could determine whether how children's teaching hospital costs differ from general acute care hospitals and whether teaching has the same effect on costs per case in children's hospitals as it has on pediatric cases in general acute care hospitals. However, we do not have the necessary cost data on children's teaching hospitals to do so. Thus, while we believe it appropriate to base the IME estimate on the costs of treating children in teaching hospitals relative to non-teaching hospitals, we cannot compare the results using this approach to one that explicitly measures IME costs in children's teaching hospitals relative to all other hospitals or other children's hospitals.

Case Mix Classification System

The case mix index should be consistent with the patient classification system selected to allocate the IME funds. That is, the patient classification system used to estimate IME should also be used to allocate IME funds under the CHGME program. For example, it would be inappropriate to use the APR-DRGs to estimate the IME effect on pediatric costs per case and the HCFA DRGs to allocate the IME funds. This is because there is an interaction between case mix and the teaching effect on cost per case. One function of the IME adjustment is to recognize severity differences that are not accounted for by the patient classification system. As more costs are explained by the patient classification system and reflected in the case mix index, the teaching variable no longer needs to account for these severity differences and has a lower coefficient.

We use the HCFA DRGs for the analyses in this report to be consistent with the HRSA decision for the FY2000 and FY2001 CHGME fund allocations. We considered using the CHAMPUS or APR-DRGs instead of the HCFA DRGs because they significantly improve the case mix classification for newborns. However, for this study we have access only to case-mix indices for children's hospitals based on HCFA DRGs. Therefore, even if we were to use a different classification system, we would not have the data for children's teaching hospitals that would allow us to use the results to simulate IME fund allocations under the CHGME program.

Relative Weights

The HCFA relative weights are based on the average cost of Medicare patients in a given DRG relative to the average cost for all Medicare patients. While in theory it would be preferable to use relative weights based on the pediatric cost data, it is not known whether this would make a significant difference in the IME estimate or in the allocation of IME funds across children's teaching hospitals. The HCFA relative weights are well-established and updated annually. In contrast, relative weights have not been established using only pediatric cases in the DRGs that are not restricted to the age 17 and under population. Utilizing the existing HCFA relative weights entails less administrative burden than establishing and maintaining pediatric relative weights. Thus, a key question for the CHGME program is whether the impact of using pediatric relative weights is sufficient to warrant developing an on-going mechanism to establish and maintain them. In this study, we investigate the relationship between relative weights based on the costs of Medicare patients and those based on the costs of pediatric patients using the HCFA DRGs. Our focus is on whether the pediatric relative weights produce a significantly different IME estimate than the HCFA relative weights. The results should inform a decision regarding whether additional analyses should be performed to determine if the pediatric relative weights would result in significantly different IME fund allocations. We do not have the DRG-level information that would allow us to use the results to simulate IME allocations to children's teaching hospitals.

Controlling for Other Explanatory Variables

Another key policy question is which variables to include in the regression equation. A fully-specified regression, which includes a comprehensive set of variables that explain differences in cost per case, provides the best technical estimate of the teaching effect. It also provides the most "technically correct" basis for allocating funds across children's teaching hospitals based solely on the indirect teaching effect. However, it may not provide the most appropriate estimate of the amounts needed to "level the playing field." This is because payers may be willing to pay higher amounts for some but not all of the other factors that have a significant effect on cost. A payer regression for the CHGME program would include as independent variables those factors that are likely to be recognized by third-party payers in purchasing care for pediatric inpatients and which do not require IME funding to "level the playing field." The decision regarding which variables to include in an IME estimate for the CHGME program is a policy decision once the set of variables that have a significant effect on cost have been identified. The decision has implications for the size of the IME coefficient. This is because teaching intensity is positively correlated with a number of the other variables. The exclusion of these variables "loads" some of their effect onto the teaching coefficient. The underlying issue is the extent to which these other factors affecting cost per case should be supported by IME funding. In this study, focus our attention in the payer regressions on those variables that are treated differently by HCFA and MedPAC. We investigate the impact that the inclusion or exclusion of the outlier and low-income variables have on the IME estimate and the allocation of IME funds across children's hospitals.

Measure of Teaching Intensity

Most resident activity is related to patient care. The resident-to-average daily census measures the relationship between the number of residents and the average number of inpatients receiving care each day and should reflect teaching intensity more directly than the resident-to-bed ratio. HCFA considers average daily census to be a better measure of teaching intensity and less subject to manipulation. It results in the same Medicare IME adjustment factor for hospitals with the same average daily census and resident count regardless of their bed size and occupancy rate (HCFA, 1991; Phillips, 1992). The MedPAC formula results in the same IME adjustment factor for hospitals with the same number of beds and resident count regardless of the number of inpatients. MedPAC prefers the resident-to-bed ratio because it favors more efficient hospitals with high occupancy rates. Relative to using the resident-to-average daily census ratio, these hospitals have a higher IME adjustment factor than hospitals with a similar resident-to average daily census ratio but lower occupancy rate.

Both the resident-to-bed ratio and resident-to-average daily census ratio are less than ideal because they relate resident activity only to inpatient services. The resident count in the numerator includes residents working in both the inpatient and outpatient areas of the hospital (as well as non-hospital settings if the hospital incurs substantially all of the training costs); therefore, it does not penalize hospitals that emphasize training in ambulatory settings. The denominator includes a measure of inpatient services only (either beds or inpatient days). In determining teaching intensity, this also advantages hospitals with a large volume of ambulatory services. They would have lower teaching intensity if the denominator included both inpatient and outpatient volume relative to a hospital with a low volume of ambulatory services and the same inpatient capacity. However, using inpatient discharges as a multiplier in the IME allocation formula penalizes hospitals with a large volume of ambulatory services. If the teaching intensity measure is adjusted for outpatient services, the multiplier should also be adjusted. In this study, we examine the effect that making both changes would have on the IME allocations across children's hospitals. In doing so, we assume that 1) a hospital's case mix index for outpatient services is comparable to its case mix index for inpatient services and 2) the teaching effect on outpatient costs is comparable to the effect on inpatient costs. Our ability to measure the teaching effect on outpatient costs is hampered by the lack of consistent measures of outpatient volume and case mix.

The way the teaching intensity variable is specified has implications for how the IME funds would be allocated across children's hospitals. The implications of the different specifications should be understood so that the choices regarding which variables are included in the regression are consistent with the policy objectives for the CHGME. It is for this reason we simulate the IME fund allocations to children's hospitals using the results from regression models with alternative measures of teaching intensity. These include not only residents-to-beds and residents-to-average daily census but also measures that take into account outpatient volume. The simulations indicate how the funds would be allocated across classes of children's teaching hospitals using alternative models that are technically appropriate. In deciding among the alternatives, the simulations provide information for determining which models are most consistent with the policy objectives for CHGME.

2. METHODS AND DATA

In the first two sub-sections below, we review our methodology for estimating an IME effect through multivariate analyses and using simulations to evaluate the sensitivity of the fund allocations to different IME estimates. We then describe the various data files that we use in our analyses. Our primary data sources are:

- 100 % claims data from 11 states participating in the Agency for Healthcare Research and Quality's Hospital Cost and Utilization Project;
- Medicare cost report data from hospitals participating in the Medicare program and filing full cost reports; and,
- HRSA-provided data reported by children's teaching hospitals during the FY2000 grant application process, including the case mix index and number of residents.

We also use information from the American Hospital Association Annual Survey to obtain data on selected facility characteristics that might explain variations in pediatric costs per case.

After we discuss our data sources, we define a series of variables that we use throughout our analyses.

ESTIMATING IME COSTS THROUGH MULTIVARIATE REGRESSION

General Specification Issues

We use multivariate regression analysis to examine various factors that may explain variation in costs per discharge across hospitals and, in particular, to estimate the effect teaching intensity has on the costs of providing care to pediatric patients. Our dependent variable is each facility's average cost per discharge. We use the natural logarithm to transform cost and to examine different specifications. Most regression models are in a log-log form. The general specification is:

$$\ln Y_i = \beta_0 + \beta_1 \ln CMI_i + \beta_2 \ln WI_i + \beta_3 \ln TI_i + \beta_4 \ln X_i + u_i$$

where:

Y = cost per discharge

CMI = the case mix index;

WI   = the area wage index

TI   = a measure of teaching intensity

X   = a vector of other variables that might affect cost
        per discharge

β = coefficients to be estimated

u = an additive error term

$_i$ = an index for each hospital

Hospital-weighted vs. discharge-weighted regressions. In preliminary analyses, we examine whether the teaching coefficients are sensitive to whether the regression is weighted. In ordinary least squares regressions, each hospital's data is given equal weight (facility-weighting). A weighted least squares estimation weights the values for each hospital by its discharges. The original Medicare IME estimates for acute care operating costs used facility-weighting. However, when this approach was used, the standard payment rate was derived from a simple average of each hospital's standardized cost per discharge. The discharge-weighted regressions should be more efficient because they give more weight to hospitals with a large number of cases. They account for the fact that there is more random variation in data from small hospitals and produce minimum variance unbiased estimates of the coefficient.

Transformation of the teaching and low-income measures. We examine different transformations of the teaching and low-income variables. These include:

- ln (1 + teaching intensity measure)
- ln (.0001 + teaching intensity measure)
- non-logged teaching intensity measure

Since the values for teaching and for serving low-income patients can be zero, [6] a customary practice has been to add 1.0 to the teaching and low-income ratios (for example, 1 + resident-to-bed ratio) before logging the variable. This form of the variable was used to estimate the original Medicare IME factor for acute care operating costs. Rogowski

_____

[6] This occurs with the teaching variable for all non-teaching hospitals. It rarely occurs for the low-income variable since at least one patient is likely to be entitled to Medicaid.

and Newhouse (1992) found that adding 1.0 to the teaching ratio biases the teaching coefficient substantially if the true specification is log-log. This is because the teaching ratios are quite small in relation to 1.0. Rogowski and Newhouse added .0001 to the teaching ratio instead of 1.0 to reduce the distortion to less than one percent. However, they also found that the revised specification did not produce a substantially different estimate of teaching hospital cost differentials. HCFA avoided the potential distortion in the ln (1 + teaching intensity measure) form by using a non-logged version of the variable in estimating the teaching effect on total costs for the capital prospective payment system (DHHS, 1991). More recently, Dalton and Norton (2000a) concluded that HCFA's original specification of the teaching variable (1+resident-to-bed ratio) is supported by the data. We examine all three forms of the teaching variable in our regressions.

Fully-Specified Regression Models

We perform a set of fully specified regressions to understand the various factors affecting costs per case and to obtain an unbiased estimate of the teaching coefficient. In most regressions, our dependent variable is the natural log of each hospital's average cost per discharge for pediatric cases. However, in some regressions we define the dependent variable as the natural log of the cost per discharge for 1) newborn (MDC 15) discharges or 2) all other discharges in order to compare how well we can explain the costs of newborns relative to other discharges. We include a comprehensive set of independent variables that may influence cost. The variables are drawn from the literature and have been shown in the past to be significant factors in explaining differences in cost per discharge across hospitals. We summarize the variables and their expected effect on cost per case in Table 1.

Table 1:	Explanatory Variables Expected to Have a Significant Effect on Cost Per Discharge	
Variable	**Definition**	**Anticipated Coefficient**
Case mix index (CMI)	The CMI measures the average resource requirements of the hospital's discharges relative to other hospitals.	The expected coefficient is 1.0.
Hospital wage index (WI)	The WI measures the average hospital hourly wage in the geographic area in which the hospital is located relative to the average hourly wage for all hospitals. About 72 percent of hospital costs are labor-related.	The expected coefficient for a variable accounting for wage-related variation (WI*.72 + .30) is 1.0.
Teaching intensity (TI)	Common measures of TI are residents-to-beds and residents-to-average daily census. Since a hospital's the resident-to-bed ratio is lower, the coefficient is higher.	While consistently significant and positive, the size depends on how TI is specified and the other variables included in the regression.
Outlier days	Outliers are typically defined as extraordinarily long-stay or costly stays within a given DRG. The variable captures patient severity that is not accounted for by the CMI. MedPAC uses the % of total Medicare payments received by a hospital that are attributable to payments for high cost outlier cases as its measure.	The coefficient is expected to be significant and positive.
Low-income patients	The measure of low-income patients typically includes the percentage of Medicaid inpatients and may also include the percentage of Medicare patients who are entitled to Supplemental Security Income. (Charity care levels are not available from public use facility-level data such as Medicare cost reports). Low-income patients tend to have more complex needs than other patients. In part, the measure serves as a proxy for patient severity that is not captured by case mix.	The coefficient is typically small and only slightly significant.
Hospital capacity	Common measures of hospital capacity are bed size, number of discharges and number of inpatient days. Larger hospitals have more infrastructure and tend to serve patients with more complex needs. On the other hand, smaller hospitals tend to be less efficient.	Indeterminate.
Emergency room admissions.	Patients admitted as emergency cases tend to have more complex needs than non-emergency patients. The variable is a measure of patient severity that is not captured by the patient classification system.	The coefficient is expected to be significant and positive.
Staffing patterns	Typical measures are staffing costs (standardized for area wage	The coefficient is expected to be

	differences) or number of full-time equivalent employees in relation to hospital capacity. Occupational mix data are not available. Larger hospitals and teaching hospitals tend to have higher staffing ratios and costs than smaller, non-teaching hospitals.	positive.
Geographic location	Dummy variables for the region in which a hospital is located was used in the original Medicare IME estimate. More recently, dummy variables for location in a large urban area and rural areas have been used (with other urban area as the missing variable) in IME estimates. Hospitals located in large urban areas tend to be larger and offer more specialized care. Rural hospitals tend to be smaller and provide less complex care. However, they also have fewer patients and higher overhead costs.	Indeterminate. Earlier studies found large urban status had a signficant effect on total cost per case. More recently, rural status has been found to have a significant effect on cost.
Type of ownership	Dummy variables are used to distinguish between hospitals by type of ownership: proprietary, non-profit, and governmental. Proprietary and governmental hospitals tend to be less costly than non-profit hospitals.	Coefficient for proprietary and/or governmental dummy variables is expected to be significant and negative.
Trauma center	A dummy variable is used to describe a hospital's status as a trauma center. The variable is used as a proxy for offering specialized services.	Coefficient for dummy variable is expected to be significant and positive.

We compare the effects of:

- using unweighted and weighted regressions;

- using CMIs derived from two different sets of relative weights: the HCFA CMI (HCFA version 16) and the Pediatric CMI (based on standardized costs for pediatric discharges); and,

- different measures of teaching intensity

Payer Regression Models

In the payer regressions, we confine our independent variables to the teaching measure and other variables that are most likely to influence the payments that hospitals receive from payers. At a minimum, the other variables are the case mix index and the wage index. We examine the effect on the teaching coefficient of including in the payer model variables for outlier cases (MedPAC approach) or low-income patients (HCFA approach) in addition to the case mix index and the wage index. Both variables are correlated with teaching activity and their inclusion or exclusion is likely to affect the teaching coefficient. We also compare the effect of using different measures of teaching intensity and logged and non-logged forms of the measures. We use the r-square and the standard error of the regression to compare the ability of the alternative models to explain variation in pediatric costs per discharge. We also use the size and significance of the wage index and case mix coefficients compared to their expected values of 1.0 as an indication of how well the model describes costs.

SIMULATING IME FUND ALLOCATIONS

We simulate allocations from the CHGME IME fund to eligible children's hospitals using the coefficients from the regression analyses. The purpose of the simulations is two-fold: to evaluate the sensitivity of the amount received by each hospital to different allocation methodologies and to estimate aggregate indirect teaching costs for the children's hospitals. The first issue analyzes the extent to which each facility's share of aggregate payments changes under different allocation policies for a fixed amount of IME funds. The second issue assesses how the different specifications affect the estimate of total IME costs changes

Our choice of IME models to simulate is designed to preserve and inform a range of policy options using HCFA CMIs. Our base model is the formula used by the Medicare program for hospital operating costs since HRSA is currently using this model to allocate IME funds. We compare the results using this model to results using Medicare's capital formula as well as results using regression coefficients derived from models based on:

- pediatric costs per case using different measures of teaching intensity
- outpatient as well as inpatient volume

Available data constrains our choice of simulations. We use the case mix index derived from the HCFA version 16 relative weights in all our simulations. We cannot simulate allocations using the case mix index that we derive from pediatric costs because we do not have case mix indices for children's teaching hospitals using these weights. Further, we do not simulate the results from regressions using outliers as an explanatory variable because we do not have information on outliers at children's hospitals.

A hospital's IME cost is a function of its case mix index (CMI), discharges, wage index, and teaching intensity. Consistent with the log-log specification, the formula for determining IME cost is multiplicative. The IME factor in the formula expresses the higher costs for teaching hospitals relative to non-teaching hospitals. Medicare IME payments are determined on a discharge-by-discharge basis and are a function of the standard payment rate adjusted for the hospital's wage index, the DRG to which the discharge is assigned, and the IME adjustment factor. Aggregate IME payments can be estimated by substituting the hospital's case mix index for the DRG relative weight and multiplying by the total number of discharges. For example, the IME adjustment factor for Medicare total costs per case using MedPAC's most recent estimate is (1+residents-to-bed ratio)$^{.31}$-1). A hospital's total Medicare IME payment under the MedPAC estimate would be:

- standard rate* CMI* (.7205*WI+ .2795) *[(1+residents-to-bed ratio)$^{.31}$-1]* number of discharges

Following this general approach, we use the coefficients from selected regressions to establish the factors that are applied to each variable. We note that the Medicare and MedPAC models assume that the coefficients for the CMI and the WI variables are 1.0. We use the actual coefficients produced by the regression to develop an allocation weighting factor (WF) for each children's teaching hospital equal to:

$$WF_i = CMI_i^{\beta cmi} * WI_i^{\beta wi} * (TI_i^{\beta ti} - 1) * (NOD_i \text{ or } NOAD_i) \text{ where:}$$

CMI_i = case mix index for hospital$_i$; βcmi= the regression coefficient for CMI

WI_i = area wage index for hospital$_i$; βwi = the regression coefficient for WI

TI_i = the teaching intensity value for hospital$_i$; βti = the regression coefficient for TI

NOD_i = number of discharges for hospital$_i$

$NOAD_i$ = number of adjusted discharges for hospital$_i$

We use the ratio of the weighting factor for the hospital to the sum of the weighting factors for all children's teaching hospitals to estimate what the hospital's share of IME funds would be. We use the coefficients from regressions using different measures of teaching intensity and forms of the measures to determine how sensitive the allocations are to the alternative formulae.

We also use the regression coefficients to estimate total IME costs in children's teaching hospitals. The estimates assume that the cost structure in children's teaching hospitals are comparable to the costs of pediatric cases in general community hospitals. They can inform the policy decision regarding the appropriate apportionment of the CHGME fund between DGME and IME. The estimates also provide information on the percentage of IME costs covered by the CHGME fund. They do not provide information on the level of coverage needed to "level the playing field."

DATA SOURCES

State Inpatient Database

The State Inpatient Database (SID) is 100% claims files maintained by the 22 states participating in the Agency for Healthcare Policy and Research's Hospital Cost and Utilization Project (HCUP). The data for 13 states are maintained centrally. Based on cost considerations, we obtain the data for 11 states to use in our analyses. The states are: Arizona, California, Colorado, Florida, Iowa, Maryland, Massachusetts, New York, Oregon, Washington, and Wisconsin. These states account for approximately 36 percent of the discharges for patients 17 and under in the United States. About 32 percent of the discharges from children's teaching hospitals occur in these States. We elect to use the SID instead of the national inpatient sample (NIS) to increase the representation of children's hospitals in our analysis file. We use the latest available information, which is for discharges occurring in 1997. We extract 2.41 million claims for patients age 17 and under. After using the AHA survey crosswalk between the AHA identification number on the claims and the Medicare provider number, we have 2.21 million discharges in our file.

Cost Report Data

We use Medicare cost report data for each Medicare participating hospital in the 11 states represented in the SID database that filed a full cost report in federal fiscal year FY 1997 (i.e., cost reporting periods beginning on or after October 1, 1996) and /or FY 1998 (i.e., cost reporting periods beginning on or after October 1, 1997). These cost reporting periods overlap the 1997 SID data. After linking the cost report data with the SID database and eliminating claims with missing charges, we have 1338 hospitals with 2.00 million discharges in our file.

Other General Hospital Data

We use other sources of information on hospital characteristics to establish explanatory variables for factors that might affect hospital costs per case. These sources are described below.

Hospital Wage Index

We obtain the hospital wage data from HCFA that were used for the FY1999 and FY2000 hospital wage indexes.

HCFA Relative Weights

We use the HCFA version 16 relative weights. These weights, which were effective for discharges occurring in FY1999, are based on FY1997 claims. They are the best match with the claims and costs data that we are using in the analysis. They are also the weights that HRSA used to allocate FY2001 IME funds.

PPS Impact File

We use HCFA's PPS impact file for FY2000. This file is made available annually when the prospective payment rates for inpatient hospital services are published. It contains the various payment parameters used to determine payments to individual acute care hospitals, such as the IME and DSH adjustments.

AHA Survey

We supplement the Medicare cost report information with data from the 1998 AHA survey on facility characteristics that might affect a hospital's cost per case. These data include: certification as a trauma center, membership in the College of Teaching Hospitals, number of fulltime equivalent employees, and adjusted average daily census. The latter variable converts outpatient services into equivalent inpatient days based on average per diem revenues.

Data on Children's Teaching Hospitals

HRSA CHGME Data

We obtain from HRSA information specific to children's hospitals that was furnished to the agency as part of the FY2000 application process for the CHGME program. The information is for 1999 and includes case mix index (HCFA version 15), number of beds, number of inpatient days and discharges, and number of FTE residents (with no weighting for residents that are beyond their initial residency period). It is more complete than the information available from Medicare cost reports since some children's teaching hospitals do not file a full Medicare cost report and case mix information is not available on the cost report.

HCUP Data

As this project was nearing completion, AHCPR obtained supplemental HCUP information from the states concerning children's inpatient stays. Summary information is available on-line and contains DRG-specific information on pediatric discharges across classes of hospitals (e.g. children's vs. general community hospitals, teaching vs. non-teaching). We use this database (KID) for information on the distribution of pediatric inpatient stays (www.ahrq.gov/hcup/hcupnet.htm).

ESTABLISHING THE VARIABLES USED IN THE ANALYSIS

Cost Per Discharge

We use the Medicare cost report data to develop for each hospital in our analysis file an overall cost-to-charge ratio for inpatient hospital services.[7] We apply the cost-to-charge ratio for inpatient

---

[7] We estimate the inpatient cost for each ancillary cost center by multiplying its total costs by the ratio of its inpatient charges to total charges. We sum the inpatient costs for the routine service areas and the ancillary areas to determine total inpatient costs and divide by total inpatient charges to develop an overall cost-to-charge ratio for

hospital services to the total charges on each SID inpatient bill for a pediatric stay to estimate the cost for the discharge. We estimate a hospital's average cost per discharge by summing the costs for all discharges in the database and dividing by the total number of discharges in the hospital. The costs include operating and capital-related costs but exclude direct medical education costs that are funded as direct GME by the Medicare and CHGME programs.

In addition to computing an average cost per discharge for all pediatric discharges at each hospital in our analysis file, we compute an average cost per discharge for the discharges assigned to MDC 15 (Newborn and other neonates with conditions originating in the perinatal period) and an average cost per discharge for patients assigned to other MDCs. We use the DRG assignment on each SID inpatient bill to separate the discharges into the appropriate groupings for these calculations.

We establish the separate cost per discharge variables for two reasons. First, the literature suggests that the HCFA DRGs do not perform well in predicting the costs of patients in MDC 15 (Averill, 1999). Second, children's teaching hospitals have a different mix of neonate cases than other hospitals. Table 2 shows the distribution of MDC 15 discharges by DRG and hospital characteristic. Sixty-eight percent of the discharges in MDC 15 are assigned to DRG 391. Children's teaching hospitals have only 9 percent of the discharges in DRG 391 compared to 12 percent of all discharges in MDC 15. They have a disproportionately large share of the discharges in DRGs for neonates with extreme prematurity or other severe problems (e.g., DRGs 386 and 387). Establishing the separate cost per discharge variables will allow us to investigate how well we are able to predict the costs for MDC 15 discharges in teaching hospitals and how the MDC 15 discharges affect our IME estimate.

Case Mix Index

We compute a CMI for each hospital in our analysis file based on HCFA version 16 relative weights. From the SID patient-level file, we

---

each hospital. After applying the cost-to-charge ratio, we adjust for inflation between the month of discharge and July 1, 1997.

Table 2: Distribution of MDC 15 Discharges By Type of Hospital

Diagnosis Related Group	N Discharges	General Community Hospital Discharges		Children's Hospital Discharges		Teaching Hospital Discharges	
		N	% of DRG Discharges	N	% of DRG Discharges	N	% of DRG Discharges
DRG 385 Neonates, died or transferred to another acute care facility	78,673	62,557	79.5%	16,116	20.5%	12,219	15.5%
DRG 386 Extreme immaturity or respiratory distress syndrome, neonate	67,897	42,272	62.3	25,625	37.70	19,878	29.3
DRG 387 Prematurity with major problems	85,715	60,515	70.6	25,199	29.4	19,791	23.1
DRG 388 Prematurity w/o major problems	126,508	102,141	80.7	24,367	19.3	19,942	15.8
DRG 389 Full term neonate with major problems	316,064	240,652	76.1	75,412	23.9	57,188	18.1
DRG 390 Neonate with other significant problems	564,290	467,409	82.8	96,881	17.2	74,082	13.1
DRG 391 Normal newborn	2,652,675	2,334,522	88.0	318,153	12.0	247,220	9.3
All MDC 15 DRGs	3,891,822	3,310,068	85.1%	581,753	14.9%	450,320	11.6%

Weighted national estimates from HCUP Kid's Inpatient Database, 1997, Agency for Healthcare Research and Quality (AHRQ), based on data collected by individual states and provided to AHRQ by the states. Total number of weighted discharges in the U.S. based on HCUP KID = 6,389,819. Note that no significance testing for differences is provided.

determine the DRG for each discharge.[8] We assign the associated relative weight for the DRG to the discharge. We determine the CMI or average relative weight by summing the hospital's relative weights and dividing by the number of discharges. In addition to an overall CMI for all the pediatric cases at each hospital, we compute separate CMIs for patients assigned to MDC 15 and other MDC s.

We use the HCFA CMI for most of our analyses since this is the only hospital-specific CMI that we have for children's teaching hospitals. We are also interested in the potential impact of using different patient classification systems and relative weights to allocate CHGME IME funds. Resource and data constraints preclude our investigating alternative patient classification systems such as the APR-DRGs for this project. However, we are able to use the claims in the SID database to establish relative weights for the HCFA DRGs that are based solely on the costs for pediatric discharges.

In developing relative weights, it is desirable to account for systematic differences in hospital mark-ups and cost levels that might affect the relative costliness of treating the average pediatric patient assigned to a given DRG compared to the average cost of pediatric patients. HCFA uses standardization to account for differences in levels

---

[8] HCUP makes the DRG assignment based on the DRG version in effect as of the date of discharge. HCFA DRG v.14 was in effect from 1/1/97-9/30/97; v.15 was in effect from 10/1/97 -12/31/97. Changes were made between the two versions in the classification logic for several DRGs. To have a consistent set of DRGs, we crosswalked the discharges from 10/1/97-12/31/97 that were assigned to the revised DRGs to the DRG they would have been assigned under v.14. The HCFA v.16 relative weights are based on Medicare discharges occurring from 10/1/96-9/30/97. We modified the relative weights to take into account DRG classification changes occurring between v. 14 and v.16 so that the weights are consistent with the v. 14 classification logic. For example, v. 15 replaced DRGs 214 and 215 (Back and neck procedures with and without CC) with 5 new DRGs: DRG 496 (Combined anterior/posterior spinal fusion), DRG 497 (Spinal fusion with CC), DRG 498 (Spinal fusion without CC) DRG 499 (Back and neck procedures except spinal fusion with CC), and DRG 500 (Back and neck procedures except spinal fusion without CC). We reassigned the pediatric discharges from the last quarter of 1997 that were classified to DRGs 497-500 to DRGs 214 and 215 based on whether they involved CCs. We also constructed relative weights for DRGs 214 and 215 using the v.16 relative weights and cases for DRGs 496-500. No changes were made over this period to DRGs with a high volume of pediatric cases.

of cost. In establishing the DRG relative weights, HCFA standardizes the hospital's charges for wage differences, teaching, and for serving low-income patients (DSH). We construct a set of relative weights using this general approach to standardize each hospital's estimated costs for a discharge. By using estimated costs rather than charges, we account for differences in overall levels of hospital mark-ups.[9]

One problem with the standardization methodology is that we need to know the teaching and low-income effect on cost in order to develop the relative weights and we need to know the average relative weight or CMI for each hospital in order to estimate the teaching and low-income patient effects. We solve this problem by using the Medicare PPS capital adjustment factors for teaching and serving a disproportionate share of low-income patients to standardize each hospital's costs per case. These factors are based on an empirical estimate of the teaching and low-income patient effect on total cost per discharge (operating and capital). For our purposes, they are preferable to the Medicare PPS operating factors since the operating factors exceed empirical estimates of the teaching and low-income effect on costs per case. We standardize the hospital's costs for the wage index as well as the capital adjustment factors.[10] We then sum the standardized cost per case for all discharges within the DRG and divide by the number of discharges within the DRG. We eliminate as statistical outliers discharges whose cost is three standard deviations or more above or below the log mean cost for the DRG. Our final analysis file has 1,337 hospitals with 1.98 million discharges.

_____

[9] Since we use an overall cost-to-charge ratio to estimate the costs for a case, we do not account for systematic differences across hospitals in mark-up policies for specific services. Applying cost-to-charge ratio specific to each ancillary department to the ancillary charges on the claim would address distortions that might exist in service mark-ups.

[10] The adjustment factors are available on the PPS impact file. To standardize, we divide the cost for each case by 1 + the sum of the IME and DSH adjustment factors. We divide the labor-related share of total costs per case by the hospital wage index. The HCFA Office of the Actuary estimates the labor-related share in FY1997 to be 72.05 percent of total costs. Standardized cost = (Cost per discharge*.7205/WI + cost per discharge*.2795)/(1+DSH+IME).

The weights we construct should be sufficient for our preliminary investigations. If we were going to use the standardized cost weights to simulate the impact pediatric-specific relative weights would have on IME allocations from the CHGME fund, we would want to develop weights through an iterative process using the coefficients from our regressions as the standardization factors. Further, we would want to compare the weights derived through standardization with weights constructed using the hospital-specific relative value method. This method converts the charges for each hospital's cases to hospital-specific relative values that are normalized for the hospital's case mix (MedPAC, 2000). Its advantage over using standardized costs is that the effect of other factors such as IME and DSH do not need to be established before developing the relative weights.

We use the relative weights to construct two case mix indices for pediatric discharges from each hospital in our database. We define the indices as follows:

- the HCFA CMI is based on the version 16 relative weights derived from Medicare discharge data; and,
- the Pediatric CMI is based on relative weights derived from pediatric discharges using the standardized cost methodology.

We develop separate case mix indices that match our cost per case variables; that is, we establish separate case mix indices for all discharges, for MDC 15 discharges and for all other discharges.

Wage Index Value

The wage index is intended to account for systematic differences in hospital wage levels across labor market areas. Medicare defines labor market areas as Metropolitan Statistical Areas (MSAs) and the non-MSA areas of States. The wage index value reflects the average hospital hourly wage in the geographic area in which a hospital is located relative to the national average hourly wage for hospitals. We use different wage indices in our regressions and in our simulations.

- In our regression analyses, we want to have the best possible match with the 1997 claims in the SID database used to derive the cost per discharge variable. We use HCFA hospital wage data for cost reporting periods beginning on or after October 1, 1996. The data were used to develop the FY2000 hospital wage index. We use the data that excludes resident and teaching physician compensation (which is defined as DGME) and classifies hospitals based on their actual geographic location without regard to reclassifications by the Medicare Geographic Reclassification Review Board.

- In our simulations of potential allocation methodologies, we use the FY1999 hospital wage index. The authorizing legislation specifies that this wage index be used to allocate direct GME funds under the CHGME program. HRSA has elected to use the same wage index to allocate the IME funds. The wage index is based on data for cost reporting periods beginning on or after October 1, 1995 and incorporates the effect of changes in geographic reclassifications.

We define the wage index as (.7205*WI +.2795). This definition takes into account that an estimated 72.05 percent of hospital total costs per discharge are labor-related.

Geographic Location

Medicare's prospective payment system recognizes geographic cost differences that are not accounted for by the hospital wage index. Specifically, there is a 1.6 percent add-on for hospitals located in a large urban area (MSAs with 1 million population or more or New England County Metropolitan Areas with 970,000 population or more) in the PPS for operating costs and a 3.0 percent add-on for capital-related costs . We establish dummy variables for location in a large urban or in a rural area to investigate whether geographic location has an effect on pediatric costs per discharge.

Hospital Capacity

We use several measures for the capacity of the hospitals in our analysis file:

- The total number of beds is a common measure of the inpatient capacity of the facility. We derive the bed size measure from

the Medicare cost report for acute care hospitals (exclusive
of sub-provider units).

- The hospital's average daily census is a measure of its
  inpatient service capacity. We derive this measure by
  dividing the total number of hospital inpatient days
  (including nursery) reported for the cost reporting period by
  the number of days in the cost reporting period.

- The hospital's adjusted average daily census is a measure of
  the total services provided by the hospital. It is determined
  by converting the hospital's outpatient services into
  equivalent inpatient days (by dividing total outpatient
  charges by the average inpatient per diem charge) and adding
  the result to inpatient days (Adj. ADC= ADC + (outpatient
  revenues/average inpatient charge per diem). The AHA survey
  data includes this variable for most hospitals. For
  children's hospitals with missing values, we impute a value.
  We multiply the hospital's ADC by the discharge-weighted
  average ratio of adjusted average daily census to average
  daily census for the hospitals for which we have both values.

Indirect Teaching Costs

We define several measures of the teaching intensity of the
hospitals in our analysis file. These include:

- Residents-to-beds based on Medicare definition. The Medicare
  PPS for operating costs uses the ratio of residents in the
  acute care portion of the facility (excluding the well
  newborn nursery) to beds (excluding well newborn nursery
  beds). Resident time spent in non-hospital settings are also
  counted if the hospital incurs substantially all of the
  costs. We use the ratio reported on the FY1999 PPS impact
  file for this variable.

- Residents-to-beds based on HRSA definition. HRSA included
  newborn nursery beds in the bed count in determining FY2001
  IME fund allocations. We construct a value by dividing total

hospital residents by the total hospital bed count reported on the cost report. [11]

- Residents-to-average daily census. This measure is used in the Medicare PPS for capital-related costs. The ratios are higher than the resident-to-bed ratio because the denominator is smaller. Relative to other hospitals with the same number of residents, hospitals with higher occupancy rates would have a lower ratio. We construct a measure from the cost report that includes well newborn nursery days.

- Residents-to-adjusted average daily census. This measure takes into account outpatient as well as inpatient services. Relative to the inpatient-only ratios, hospitals with a higher proportion of outpatient services would have a lower ratio.

Low-Income Patients

We establish a low-income patient measure for each hospital based on the proportion of total pediatric inpatient days that are attributable to Medicaid patients. The low- income patient measure accounts for additional patient severity and other costs associated with serving low-income patients. It is not a measure of the facility's uncompensated care costs.

Outlier Stays

We develop a measure of the percentage of each facility's inpatient days that are attributable to atypically long lengths of stay. The measure is a way of accounting for severity of illness that is not accounted for by the case mix index. We develop the measure by establishing an outlier threshold for each DRG as the mean length of stay plus one standard deviation for the cases assigned to the DRG. We define the outlier value for each facility the percentage of its inpatient days that exceed the DRG-specific outlier thresholds. In addition to an overall measure for all discharges, we develop separate

---

[11] From the Medicare cost report, we divide Worksheet S-3, Part I, Line 12, Column 7 by Worksheet S-3, Part I, line 12, Column 1.

outlier percentages for MDC 15 discharges only and for all other discharges.

Percent Admissions from Emergency Room

We use the source of admission data on the SID claims to estimate the percentage of admissions that occur through the emergency room. We use this measure as an explanatory variable in the full-specified regressions. Patients who are admitted through the emergency room tend to have a higher cost per discharge than other patients.

Ratio of Employees to Adjusted Average Daily Census

We use the AHA survey data to compute the ratio of full-time employees on the hospital staff to the hospital's adjusted average daily census. The ratio provides a measure of the size of the hospital's staff in relation to its patient load. We use the measure as an explanatory variable in the full-specified regressions. Teaching hospitals tend to have a higher staffing ratio than other hospitals.

3. ANALYSIS RESULTS

FACILITY CHARACTERISTICS

Table 3 summarizes key characteristics of the hospitals in our analysis file and compares them to the universe of general acute care hospitals and children's teaching hospitals. In total, there are 1337 hospitals in the analysis file, of which 958 are non-teaching and 370 are teaching. These are hospitals for which we were able to link the SID database with Medicare cost report data. We chose to use the HCUP SID database over the 20% national sample of hospitals in the expectation that it would allow us to include data for children's teaching hospitals in our analysis file. However, there were only 8 children's hospitals in the SID database for the 11 states included in the file. After linking the SID data with Medicare cost report data, we were able to determine the average cost per discharge for only two children's hospitals. Therefore, children's hospitals are significantly under-represented in the analysis file used for the regression analyses and are not separately reported. We separately report the data for teaching hospitals based on membership in the College of Teaching Hospitals. Relative to non-COTH hospitals, COTH members are larger, treat children with more complex needs, and have larger residency training programs.

We use information on from the Medicare PPS impact file to compare the hospitals in the analysis file with the characteristics of the universe of general acute care hospitals.

- Compared to the universe, a higher proportion of hospitals is located in large urban areas and a lower proportion is located in rural areas. This distribution explains the higher average wage index for the hospitals in the analysis file (1.0307 vs. .9378).
- Overall, the hospitals in the analysis file are also somewhat larger.
  - o The average daily census is 98 patients compared to 87 patients in the hospital universe.

Table 3: Comparison of Hospitals in Analysis File with Universe of General Community Hospitals and Children's Teaching

	HOSPITALS IN ANALYSIS FILE					GENERAL ACUTE CARE HOSPITALS		
	All	Non Teaching	Teaching	COTH	Non COTH	All	Non- Teaching	Teaching
General Facility Characteristics								
Number of Hospitals	1337	958	370	89	281	5,070	3955	1115
% Large Urban	47	37	71	84	66	33	24	61
% Other Urban	24	24	25	13	28	24	21	33
% Rural	30	40	5	2	6	44	55	5
Average Number of Beds	188	134	333	551	264	145	102	299
% Certified Trauma Centers	26	22	37	51	32			
Average Daily Census	98	60	192	351	141	87	46	192
Adjusted Average Daily Census	185	129	332	576	255			
Average Hospital Wage Index Value	1.0307	1.0032	1.0953	1.1422	1.0804	0.9378	0.9111	1.0327
Teaching Status								
Average No. of Residents			76	235	26			72
Resident-to-Bed Ratio			0.177	0.427	0.097			0.191
Resident-to-Average Daily Census Ratio			0.300	0.670	0.183			0.316
Resident-to-Adjusted Average Daily Census Ratio			0.175	0.408	0.101			missing

CHILDREN'S TEACHING HOSPITALS

General Facility Characteristics	All	Non Teaching	Teaching	COTH	Non COTH
Number of Facilities	55		55	18	37
% Large Urban	78		78	89	73
% Other Urban	22		22	11	27
% Rural	0		0	0	0
Average Number of Beds	182		182	213	166
% Certified Trauma Centers	62		62	83	51
Average Daily Census	124		124	148	136
Adjusted Average Daily Census	186		186	228	205
Average Hospital Wage Index Value	1.0287		1.0287	1.0191	1.0333
Teaching Status					
Average No. of Residents	79		79	135	52
Resident-to-Bed Ratio	0.384		0.384	0.592	0.282
Resident-to-Average Daily Census Ratio	0.581		0.581	0.872	0.439
Resident-to-Adjusted Average Daily Census Ratio	0.389		0.389	0.572	0.300

Table 4: Distribution of Pediatric Discharges Across High Volume Diagnosis- Related Groups in All Hospitals Compared to Hospitals in Analysis File

DRG No.	Diagnosis Related Group Name	ALL HOSPITALS[1]		HOSPITALS IN ANALYSIS FILE		
		Rank	Discharges N	Rank	Discharges N	% of All DRG Discharges
391	Normal newborn	1	2,652,675	1	935,970	35.3%
390	Neonate w other significant problems	2	564,290	2	189,769	33.6%
98	Bronchitis & asthma age 0-17	3	354,395	4	87,892	24.8%
389	Full term neonate w major problems	4	316,064	3	101,739	32.2%
91	Simple pneumonia & pleurisy age 0-17	5	184,451	6	44,033	23.9%
184	Esophagitis, gastroent & misc digest disorders age 0-17	6	162,989	8	39,374	24.2%
373	Vaginal delivery w/o complicating diagnoses	7	138,890	5	44,205	31.8%
388	Prematurity w/o major problems	8	126,508	7	40,039	31.6%
298	Nutritional & misc metabolic disorders age 0-17	9	105,669	10	26,676	25.2%
387	Prematurity w major problems	10	85,715	9	28,076	32.8%
422	Viral illness & fever of unknown origin age 0-17	11	80,248	12	19,731	24.6%
385	Neonates, died or transfer to another acute care facility	12	78,673	11	23,102	29.4%
386	Extreme immaturity or respiratory distress syndrome, neonate	13	67,897	13	19,599	28.9%
430	Psychoses	14	66,099	16	14,893	22.5%
6	Seizure & headache age 0-17	15	62,000	14	15,864	25.6%
0	Otitis media & URI age 0-17	16	51,784	17	12,728	24.6%
22	Kidney & urinary tract infections age 0-17	17	48,547	18	12,633	26.0%
67	Appendectomy w/o complicated principal diag w/o CC	18	44,878	15	15,320	34.1%
451	Poisoning & toxic effects of drugs age 0-17	19	33,521	19	9,290	27.7%
79	Cellulitis age 0-17	20	30,268	20	7,987	26.4%
17	Septicemia age 0-17	21	29,217	23	7,173	24.6%
96	Red blood cell disorders age 0-17	22	29,179	26	6,785	23.3%
1	Laryngotracheitis	23	28,176	22	7,349	26.1%
431	Childhood mental disorders	24	27,693	24	6,978	25.2%
295	Diabetes age 0-35	25	26,733	27	5,939	22.2%
220	Lower extrem & humer proc except hip, foot,femur age 0-17	26	25,390	21	7,575	29.8%
410	Chemotherapy w/o acute leukemia as secondary diagnosis	27	25,341	28	5,713	22.5%
3	Craniotomy age 0-17	28	24,696	30	5,455	22.1%

DRG	Description				
372	Vaginal delivery w complicating diagnoses	29	24,409	25	6,845	28.0%
212	Hip & femur procedures except major joint age 0-17	30	19,932	31	5,048	25.3%
30	Traumatic stupor & coma, coma	31	19,330	29	5,614	29.0%
426	Depressive neuroses	32	18,368	33	4,730	25.8%
33	Viral meningitis	33	16,217	34	4,614	28.5%
90	Other digestive system diagnoses age 0-17	34	15,961	36	4,225	26.5%
156	Stomach, esophageal & duodenal procedures age 0-17	35	15,834	37	3,818	24.1%
371	Cesarean section w/o CC	36	15,063	32	4,786	31.8%
165	Appendectomy w complicated principal diag w/o CC	37	13,645	35	4,554	33.4%
108	Other cardiothoracic procedures	38	13,313	43	2,729	20.5%
81	Respiratory infections & inflammations age 0-17	39	13,282	39	3,378	25.4%
475	Respiratory system diagnosis with ventilator support	40	12,318	41	3,110	25.2%
83	Other antepartum diagnoses w medical complications	41	12,198	38	3,522	28.9%
92	Chemotherapy w acute leukemia as secondary diagnosis	42	11,988	46	2,629	21.9%
398	Reticuloendothelial & immunity disorders w CC	3	11,287	47	2,498	22.1%
427	Neuroses except depressive	44	10,540	40	3,242	30.8%
370	Cesarean section w CC	5	10,226	44	2,691	26.3%
470	Ungroupable	46	9,679			0.0%
255	Fx, sprn, strn & disl of uparm, lowleg ex foot age 0-17	47	9,572	42	3,082	32.2%
20	Nervous system infection except viral meningitis	48	9,523	48	2,488	26.1%
468	Extensive O.R. procedure unrelated to principal diagnosis	49	9,164	52	2,352	25.7%
60	Tonsillectomy &/or adenoidectomy only, age 0-17	50	8,979	57	2,079	23.2%
97	Coagulation disorders	51	8915		2,351	26.4%

Total Discharges in Top 50 DRGs 5,722,814 1,823,017 31.9%

Discharges in Other DRGS 667,005 158,292 23.7%

TOTAL DISCHARGES 6,389,819 1,981,309 31.0%

[1]Weighted national estimates from HCUP Kid's Inpatient Database, 1997, Agency for Healthcare Research and Quality (AHRQ), based on data collected by individual states and provided to AHRQ by the states. Total number of weighted discharges in the U.S.based on HCUP KID=6,389,819.

o Non-teaching hospitals in the analysis file have an average daily census of 60 patients vs. 46 patients in the universe.

o The average daily census for teaching hospitals is the same in both the analysis file and the universe (192 patients).

We also use the information we have obtained on children's teaching hospitals to compare them to the hospitals in our analysis file.

- The children's teaching hospitals tend to be smaller, with an average daily census of 124 patients. The COTH children's teaching hospitals have an average daily census of 148 patients compared to 351 patients for the general teaching hospitals in our analysis file.

- The average number of residents is comparable. The children's teaching hospitals have 76 residents on average compared to an average of 79 residents for the hospitals in the analysis file.

- With smaller patient loads, the children's hospitals have substantially higher teaching intensity ratios. The average ratio of residents-to-average daily census is .581 for children's teaching hospitals compared to .300 for the hospitals in the analysis file.

DISCHARGE CHARACTERISTICS

Table 4 shows the percentage of discharges in high-volume DRGs that are accounted for in our analysis file.

- In total, there are 1,981,309 discharges, of which 92 percent are in the top 50 DRGs by volume.

- The file accounts for 31.0 percent of all discharges, 31.9 percent of the discharges in the high-volume DRGs, and 23.7 percent of the remaining discharges. By DRG, the range is from a high of 35.3 percent in DRG 391 (Normal newborn) to 20.2 percent in DRG 108 (Other cardio-thoracic procedures).

- There are some DRGs with a large number of discharges that are underrepresented. For example, the file accounts for

24.8% and 23.9%, respectively, of the estimated discharges in DRG 98 (Bronchitis and asthma age 0-17) and DRG 91 (Simple pneumonia and pleurisy age 0-17).

- Overall, the DRGs in MDC 15 are over-represented relative to the DRGs in other MDCs. Since the average relative weight is lower for MDC 15 discharges than discharges in other DRGs, it is likely that the average CMI for the hospitals in the analysis file is somewhat lower than the average CMI for pediatric cases across all hospitals.

Table 5 summarizes the characteristics of the pediatric cases across the classes of teaching hospitals in our analysis file. Teaching hospitals generally (and COTH members to a greater extent) are larger, have a lower proportion of discharges in MDC 15, a higher case mix and longer length of stay.

- The teaching hospitals have on average 2,785 pediatric discharges compared to an average of 945 discharges in the non-teaching hospitals. The COTH hospitals have more than twice the number of discharges (4,695) than the other teaching hospitals in the analysis file.

- About 57 percent of the pediatric discharges in COTH hospitals occur in MDC 15 compared to 68 percent of the discharges in other teaching hospitals and 73 percent in non-teaching hospitals.

- Reflecting the higher case mix, the average length of stay in COTH hospitals is 4.3 days compared to 3.1 in non-COTH teaching hospitals and 2.3 days in non-teaching hospitals.

- The HCFA v.16 average relative weight for the pediatric discharges across all hospitals in the analysis file is .7539. The HCFA CMI in teaching hospitals is .8423 compared to .6419 in non-teaching hospitals.

Table 5: Characteristics of Pediatric Discharges by Classes of Hospital in Analysis File

HOSPITALS IN ANALYSIS FILE

	All	Non Teaching	Teaching	COTH	Non COTH
No. of Hospitals	1,337	958	370	89	281
Average No. of Pediatric Discharges	1,482	945	2,785	4,695	2,180
MDC15	1,001	687	1,779	2,685	1,493
Other MDCs	481	258	1,006	2,010	688
Average Length of Stay (days)	3.1	2.4	3.6	4.3	3.2
MDC15	2.9	2.3	3.4	4.3	3.1
Other MDCs	3.6	2.9	3.8	4.4.	3.6
HCFA v.16 CMI	0.7539	0.6419	0.8423	0.9623	0.7604
Standardized HCFA V.16 CMI	1.0000	0.8515	1.1172	1.2764	1.0086
MDC15	0.9138	0.7948	1.0302	1.1758	0.9472
Other MDCs	1.2052	1.0190	1.3015	1.4462	1.1676
Pediatric Case Mix Index	1.0000	0.7756	1.1719	1.4049	1.0129
MDC15	0.7625	0.5951	0.9167	1.1183	0.8019
Other MDCs	1.5439	1.2654	1.6931	1.8775	1.5225
% Pediatric Outlier Days	10.8	7	12.3	15.1	10.5
% Medicaid Discharges	38.1	37.1	38.7	39.8	37.9
Costs					
Average Cost per Case	$2,012	$1,597	$3,498	$5,230	$2,317
MDC15	$1,316	$799	$2,909	$5,115	$1,653
Other MDCs	$2,887	$2,507	$4,428	$5,790	$3,167
No. of FTEs per adjusted ADC	4.6	4.0	5.0	6.0	4.7

To facilitate case mix comparisons, we normalize the relative weights so that the average HCFA relative weight for the discharges in our analysis file is 1.0.[12]

- The normalized CMI for the MDC 15 discharges is .9138, or slightly more than 8 percent lower than the average relative weight.

- The normalized CMI for non-MDC 15 discharges is 1.2052, or about 20.5 percent higher than the average relative weight for all discharges in the analysis file.

- The CMI for discharges from teaching hospitals is about 11 percent higher than average while the CMI for discharges from non-teaching hospitals discharges is about 15 percent lower than average.

- The CMI for COTH hospitals is about 28 percent higher than the average CMI for all pediatric discharges and for discharges from other teaching hospitals.

The pediatric relative weights constructed from standardized pediatric costs per discharge produce relatively lower CMIs for MDC 15 discharges and relatively higher CMIs for non-MDC 15 discharges. This suggests that the HCFA relative weights understate the relative complexity of non-MDC15 discharges.

- The CMI for the MDC15 discharges drops from .9138 to .7625.
- The CMI for non-MDC 15 discharges increases from 1.2052 to 1.5439.

The pediatric relative weights provide greater differentiation in the case mix across classes of teaching hospitals.

- The CMI for the discharges from COTH hospitals are 40 percent higher than the average relative weight for all discharges (compared to 28 percent using the HCFA CMIs).

- The COTH hospitals also have the highest percentage of outlier days: 15.1 percent compared to 10.8 percent across all discharges.

---

[12] To normalize, we divide each relative weight (or case mix index) by .7539.

Table 6: High Volume DRGs in Analysis File Number of Discharge, Average Length of Stay, Outlier Thresholds and Percent Outlier Days

DRG	DC	DRG Name	N Discharges	% of Discharges in Analysis File	Average Length of Stay	Outlier Threshold	Outlier Days as Percent of Total DRG Days
391	15	NORMAL NEWBORN	935970	47.24%	1.75	2.66	6.38
390	15	NEONATE W OTHER SIGNIFICANT PROBLEMS	189769	9.58%	2.26	3.83	7.54
389	15	FULL TERM NEONATE W MAJOR PROBLEMS	101739	5.13%	4.19	9.00	13.30
98	4	BRONCHITIS & ASTHMA AGE 0-17	87892	4.44%	2.69	4.53	8.31
373	14	VAGINAL DELIVERY W/O COMPLICATING DIAGNOSES	44205	2.23%	1.79	2.93	4.47
91	4	SIMPLE PNEUMONIA & PLEURISY AGE 0-17	44033	2.22%	3.24	5.51	8.48
388	15	PREMATURITY W/O MAJOR PROBLEMS	40039	2.02%	4.62	9.70	16.35
184	6	ESOPHAGITIS	39374	1.99%	2.27	4.29	9.49
387	15	PREMATURITY W MAJOR PROBLEMS	28076	1.42%	14.98	29.44	12.89
298	10	NUTRITIONAL & MISC METABOLIC DISORDERS AGE 0-17	26676	1.35%	2.58	5.04	12.32
385	15	NEONATES	23102	1.17%	4.93	18.44	38.25
422	18	VIRAL ILLNESS & FEVER OF UNKNOWN ORIGIN AGE 0-17	19731	1.00%	2.62	4.27	6.85
386	15	EXTREME IMMATURITY OR RESPIRATORY DISTRESS SYNDROME	19599	0.99%	33.88	66.31	12.86
26	1	SEIZURE & HEADACHE AGE 0-17	15864	0.80%	2.57	5.17	11.50
167	6	APPENDECTOMY W/O COMPLICATED PRINCIPAL DIAG W/O CC	15320	0.77%	2.07	3.23	6.18
430	19	PSYCHOSES	14893	0.75%	8.58	18.06	13.27
70	3	OTITIS MEDIA & URI AGE 0-17	12728	0.64%	2.52	4.24	7.68
322	11	KIDNEY & URINARY TRACT INFECTIONS AGE 0-17	12633	0.64%	3.57	5.82	7.49
451	21	POISONING & TOXIC EFFECTS OF DRUGS AGE 0-17	9290	0.47%	1.72	3.44	11.84
279	9	CELLULITIS AGE 0-17	7987	0.40%	3.08	5.08	8.01
220	8	LOWER EXTREM & HUMER PROC EXCEPT HIP	7575	0.38%	2.12	4.27	11.27
71	3	LARYNGOTRACHEITIS	7349	0.37%	1.61	2.79	8.56
417	18	SEPTICEMIA AGE 0-17	7173	0.36%	4.38	7.76	10.19
431	19	CHILDHOOD MENTAL DISORDERS	6978	0.35%	9.65	20.09	14.00
372	14	VAGINAL DELIVERY W COMPLICATING DIAGNOSES	6845	0.35%	2.58	4.89	8.88
396	16	RED BLOOD CELL DISORDERS AGE 0-17	6785	0.34%	3.97	7.54	11.42
295	10	DIABETES AGE 0-35	5939	0.30%	3.05	5.47	8.58
410	17	CHEMOTHERAPY W/O ACUTE LEUKEMIA AS SECONDARY DIAGNOSIS	5713	0.29%	3.32	5.58	6.36
30	1	TRAUMATIC STUPOR & COMA	5614	0.28%	2.11	4.79	13.54

3	1	CRANIOTOMY AGE 0-17	5455	0.28%	8.22	19.49	17.70
212	8	HIP & FEMUR PROCEDURES EXCEPT MAJOR JOINT AGE 0-17	5048	0.25%	4.39	9.44	16.11
371	14	CESAREAN SECTION W/O CC	4786	0.24%	3.43	5.52	4.93
426	19	DEPRESSIVE NEUROSES	4730	0.24%	5.96	12.77	13.19
21	1	VIRAL MENINGITIS	4614	0.23%	3.13	5.36	9.10
165	6	APPENDECTOMY W COMPLICATED PRINCIPAL DIAG W/O CC	4554	0.23%	4.68	7.18	5.74
190	6	OTHER DIGESTIVE SYSTEM DIAGNOSES AGE 0-17	4225	0.21%	2.83	7.39	18.54
156	6	STOMACH, ESOPHAGEAL & DUODENAL PROCEDURES AGE 0-17	3818	0.19%	5.66	14.30	18.88
383	14	OTHER ANTEPARTUM DIAGNOSES W MEDICAL COMPLICATIONS	3522	0.18%	2.68	5.59	9.97
81	4	RESPIRATORY INFECTIONS & INFLAMMATIONS AGE 0-17	3378	0.17%	6.81	12.78	10.78
427	19	NEUROSES EXCEPT DEPRESSIVE	3242	0.16%	6.44	14.11	14.08
475	4	RESPIRATORY SYSTEM DIAGNOSIS WITH VENTILATOR SUPPORT	3110	0.16%	10.26	20.44	13.12
255	8	FX, SPRN, STRN & DISL OF UPARM, LOWLEG EX FOOT AGE 0-17	3082	0.16%	1.62	3.10	10.71
108	5	OTHER CARDIOTHORACIC PROCEDURES	2729	0.14%	9.32	18.03	13.36
370	14	CESAREAN SECTION W CC	2691	0.14%	4.69	8.05	7.91
282	9	TRAUMA TO THE SKIN	2676	0.14%	1.41	2.85	11.25
492	17	CHEMOTHERAPY W ACUTE LEUKEMIA AS SECONDARY DIAGNOSIS	2629	0.13%	3.33	5.71	8.36
398	16	RETICULOENDOTHELIAL & IMMUNITY DISORDERS W CC	2498	0.13%	5.25	10.13	11.63
20	1	NERVOUS SYSTEM INFECTION EXCEPT VIRAL MENINGITIS	2488	0.13%	7.19	13.37	10.29
379	14	THREATENED ABORTION	2434	0.12%	2.82	7.07	19.43
33	1	CONCUSSION AGE 0-17	2417	0.12%	1.27	2.13	8.12
164	6	APPENDECTOMY W COMPLICATED PRINCIPAL DIAG W CC	2372	0.12%	7.21	11.23	7.00
		Total Discharges in Top 50 DRGs	1823017	92.01%			

These findings indicate that on average COTH members serve more severely ill patients than other hospitals.

In Table 6, we present DRG-specific information on the discharges in the analysis file. The top 50 DRGs in volume (which account for 92 percent of the discharges in our analysis file) are arrayed in descending order by number of discharges. The average length of stay for the discharges assigned to each DRG is shown as well as the outlier threshold used to determine the percentage of days that are more than one standard deviation above the mean length of stay for the DRG. Most DRGs have an average length of stay that is less than 3 days. A high percentage of outlier days indicates that the DRG classification system may not be capturing systematic differences in severity within the DRG. In this regard, we note that several MDC 15 DRGs have a disproportionately high percentage of outlier days (for example, DRG 389, 13.3%; DRG 388, 16.35%; and, DRG 385, 38.25%). This finding is consistent with findings from earlier studies that the HCFA DRGs do not predict costs well for neonate discharges. Also, the DRGs related to mental disorders (MDC 19) have consistently higher outlier day percentages[13].

RELATIVE WEIGHT COMPARISON

In Table 7, we report DRG-specific information pertaining to the relative weights used to construct the case mix indices for the hospitals in our analysis file. The standardized cost per discharge is the average cost for pediatric discharges assigned to the DRG after standardization using the FY2000 hospital wage index and the payment parameters for IME and DSH used under the Medicare capital prospective payment system.

- The pediatric relative weight for each DRG is based on the ratio of the average standardized cost for the discharges in the DRG relative to the average standardized cost for all

---

[13] In this regard, we note that psychiatric hospitals and units are excluded from the Medicare prospective payment system because of the inability to develop to date an adequate case mix classification system for psychiatric stays.

Table 7: High Volume DRGs Standardized Cost Per Discharge and Comparison of HFCA and Pediatric Relative Weights

DRG	N Discharges	DRG Name	Standardized Cost Per Case	Pediatric Relative Weight	HCFA v.16 Relative Weight	Normalized HCFA Relative Weight	Normalized Pediatric RW	Ratio of Pediatric RW to HCFA Normalized RW
390	189769	NEONATE W OTHER SIGNIFICANT PROBLEMS	824	0.3741	1.5908	2.1102		0.18
492	2629	CHEMOTHERAPY W ACUTE LEUKEMIA AS SECONDARY DIAGNOSIS	3211	1.4571	4.5427	6.0258		0.24
388	40039	PREMATURITY W/O MAJOR PROBLEMS	2346	1.0647	1.8578	2.4643		0.43
396	6785	RED BLOOD CELL DISORDERS AGE 0-17	3106	1.4096	2.1978	2.9153		0.48
389	101739	FULL TERM NEONATE W MAJOR PROBLEMS	2805	1.2729	1.8279	2.4247		0.53
21	4614	VIRAL MENINGITIS	2403	1.0904	1.4753	1.9569		0.56
71	7349	LARYNGOTRACHEITIS	1305	0.5923	0.783	1.0386		0.57
20	2488	NERVOUS SYSTEM INFECTION EXCEPT VIRAL MENINGITIS	6093	2.7650	2.6102	3.4624		0.80
417	7173	SEPTICEMIA AGE 0-17	3099	1.4063	1.3276	1.7610		0.80
184	39374	ESOPHAGITIS	1620	0.7352	0.5457	0.7239		1.02
298	26676	NUTRITIONAL & MISC METABOLIC DISORDERS AGE 0-17	1575	0.7148	0.5262	0.6980		1.02
391	935970	NORMAL NEWBORN	456	0.2069	0.1516	0.2011		1.03
98	87892	BRONCHITIS & ASTHMA AGE 0-17	2116	0.9602	0.6953	0.9223		1.04
295	5939	DIABETES AGE 0-35	2278	1.0338	0.7242	0.9606		1.08
108	2729	OTHER CARDIOTHORACIC PROCEDURES	18954	8.6013	5.9764	7.9275		1.09
279	7987	CELLULITIS AGE 0-17	2128	0.9657	0.6627	0.8791		1.10
422	19731	VIRAL ILLNESS & FEVER OF UNKNOWN ORIGIN AGE 0-17	1838	0.8341	0.5668	0.7518		1.11
26	15864	SEIZURE & HEADACHE AGE 0-17	2395	1.0866	0.7277	0.9653		1.13
167	15320	APPENDECTOMY W/O COMPLICATED PRINCIPAL DIAG W/O CC	2924	1.3268	0.8522	1.1304		1.17
91	44033	SIMPLE PNEUMONIA & PLEURISY AGE 0-17	2549	1.1566	0.7209	0.9563		1.21
190	4225	OTHER DIGESTIVE SYSTEM DIAGNOSES AGE 0-17	2680	1.2160	0.7519	0.9974		1.22
387	28076	PREMATURITY W MAJOR PROBLEMS	11375	5.1618	3.0791	4.0843		1.26
373	44205	VAGINAL DELIVERY W/O COMPLICATING DIAGNOSES	1561	0.7082	0.4	0.5306		1.33
398	2498	RETICULOENDOTHELIAL & IMMUNITY DISORDERS W CC	4870	2.2101	1.2463	1.6532		1.34
165	4554	APPENDECTOMY W COMPLICATED PRINCIPAL DIAG W/O CC	4797	2.1767	1.2269	1.6274		1.34
81	3378	RESPIRATORY INFECTIONS & INFLAMMATIONS AGE 0-17	5910	2.6821	1.5098	2.0027		1.34
372	6845	VAGINAL DELIVERY W COMPLICATING DIAGNOSES	2287	1.0380	0.5716	0.7582		1.37
370	2691	CESAREAN SECTION W CC	4303	1.9529	1.0501	1.3929		1.40

322	12633	KIDNEY & URINARY TRACT INFECTIONS AGE 0-17	2249	1.0206	0.5406	0.7171	1.42
475	3110	RESPIRATORY SYSTEM DIAGNOSIS WITH VENTILATOR SUPPORT	15686	7.1184	3.7429	4.9648	1.43
383	3522	OTHER ANTEPARTUM DIAGNOSES W MEDICAL COMPLICATIONS	2035	0.9234	0.4718	0.6258	1.48
371	4786	CESAREAN SECTION W/O CC	3211	1.4571	0.7161	0.9499	1.53
430	14893	PSYCHOSES	3661	1.6614	0.8079	1.0717	1.55
379	2434	THREATENED ABORTION	1995	0.9055	0.439	0.5823	1.55
410	5713	CHEMOTHERAPY W/O ACUTE LEUKEMIA AS SECONDARY DIAGNOSIS	3831	1.7384	0.8402	1.1145	1.56
70	12728	OTITIS MEDIA & URI AGE 0-17	1843	0.8365	0.3841	0.5095	1.64
426	4730	DEPRESSIVE NEUROSES	2659	1.2065	0.5525	0.7329	1.65
385	23102	NEONATES	6824	3.0965	1.3671	1.8134	1.71
427	3242	NEUROSES EXCEPT DEPRESSIVE	2895	1.3140	0.5588	0.7412	1.77
431	6978	CHILDHOOD MENTAL DISORDERS	4130	1.8743	0.7468	0.9906	1.89
220	7575	LOWER EXTREM & HUMER PROC EXCEPT HIP	3691	1.6751	0.5803	0.7698	2.18
3	5455	CRANIOTOMY AGE 0-17	12407	5.6303	1.9449	2.5799	2.18
255	3082	FX, SPRN, STRN & DISL OF UPARM, LOWLEG EX FOOT AGE 0-17	2061	0.9355	0.2935	0.3893	2.40
212	5048	HIP & FEMUR PROCEDURES EXCEPT MAJOR JOINT AGE 0-17	5959	2.7043	0.8413	1.1160	2.42
451	9290	POISONING & TOXIC EFFECTS OF DRUGS AGE 0-17	1861	0.8444	0.2614	0.3467	2.44
156	3818	STOMACH, ESOPHAGEAL & DUODENAL PROCEDURES AGE 0-17	6227	2.8257	0.8378	1.1113	2.54
33	2417	CONCUSSION AGE 0-17	1600	0.7259	0.2072	0.2748	2.64
386	19599	EXTREME IMMATURITY OR RESPIRATORY DISTRESS SYNDROME	34897	15.8361	4.5084	5.9803	2.65
30	5614	TRAUMATIC STUPOR & COMA	2565	1.1641	0.3297	0.4373	2.66
282	2676	TRAUMA TO THE SKIN	2157	0.9786	0.2552	0.3385	2.89

- discharges. Thus, the average pediatric relative weight is 1.0.
- A discharge assigned to a DRG with a relative weight of 1.10 is on average 10 percent more costly than the average pediatric discharge while a discharge assigned to a DRG with a relative weight of .85 is 15 percent less costly on average.

We compare the pediatric relative weight to the HCFA v.16 relative weights. As indicated earlier, the average HCFA relative weight for pediatric cases is .7539. To facilitate the comparison between the two sets of relative weights, we normalize the HCFA relative weights by dividing each DRG weight by .7539 so that the average HCFA relative weight after normalization is also 1.0. We then divide the pediatric relative weight by the normalized HCFA relative weight to summarize their relationship.

We array the DRGs in the table in ascending order of the ratios of the pediatric relative weights to the normalized HCFA relative weights. We find that there are substantial differences in the two sets of relative weights that could have marked impact of the allocation of IME funds across children's teaching hospitals. Of concern are those DRGs at either extreme.

- DRG 390 (Neonates with other major problems), which has the second highest number of cases, has the lowest ratio. The pediatric relative weight for DRG 390 is only 18 percent of the normalized HCFA relative weight.
- The pediatric relative weight for DRG 386 (Extreme immaturity or respiratory distress syndrome) is more than 2.65 times greater than the normalized HCFA relative weight. Since DRG 386 carries a high weight, the absolute differences are large as well: 15.84 versus 4.51.

The HCFA relative weights for these MDC 15 DRGs were constructed originally from pediatric data. We expected the HCFA and pediatric

					EXPLANATORY VARIABLES (WI in ALL)			
Table	Model	Type	Discharges in Cost Per Case	CMI	Teaching Measure	Outlier	Low-Income Patient	Other
9	A	F/S	All	HCFA	ln(1+R2ADC)	√	√	√
	B	F/S	All- No Wgt	HCFA	ln(1+R2ADC)	√	√	√
	C	F/S	All	HCFA	ln(1+R2Beds)	√	√	√
	D	F/S	All	PED	ln(1+R2ADC)	√	√	√
10	A	F/S	All	HCFA	ln(1+R2DC)	√	√	√
		F/S	No MDC15	HCFA	ln(1+R2ADC)	√	√	√
		F/S	MDC 15	HCFA	ln(1+R2ADC)	√	√	√
11	1	Pay	All	HCFA	ln(1+R2ADC)			
	2	Pay	All	HCFA	ln(1+R2Beds)			
	3	Pay	All	HCFA	ln(1+R2AdjADC)			
	4	Pay	All	HCFA	ln(1+ FTE resident)			
12	5	Pay	All	HCFA	ln(1+R2ADC)	√		
	6	Pay	All	HCFA	ln(1+R2ADC)		√	
A12*	5	Pay	All	HCFA	ln(1+R2ADC)	√		
		Pay	All	HCFA	ln(1+R2Beds)	√		
		Pay	All	HCFA	ln(1+R2AdjADC)	√		
		Pay	All	HCFA	ln(1+ FTE resident)	√		
13	5	Pay	All	HCFA	ln(1+R2ADC)	√		
	5A	Pay	All	HCFA	ln(.0001+R2ADC)	√		
	5B	Pay	All	HCFA	Non-log R2ADC	√		
14	5	Pay	All	HCFA	ln(1+R2ADC)	√		
		Pay	No MDC15	HCFA	ln(1+R2ADC)	√		
		Pay	MDC 15	HCFA	ln(1+R2ADC)	√		
		Pay	No MDC15	PED	ln(1+R2ADC)	√		
		Pay	MDC 15	PED	ln(1+R2ADC)	√		

Table 8: Overview of Regression Models Included in Report Tables

*Appendix

relative weights for the MDC-15 DRGs to be more similar than those constructed largely with Medicare claims data. Further analysis is needed to determine why there are such marked differences in some of the DRGs. One reason may be that we are using an overall cost-to-charge ratio to determine per discharge costs. Historically, hospitals have had lower markups for maternity care than other inpatient care. This would tend to understate the cost of these cases relative to non-maternity cases. With regard to DRG 390, it may be that coding practices have led to the more complex cases being assigned to a higher weighted DRG. As seen in Table 6, DRG 390 has a relatively low outlier threshold and percentage of outlier days, which indicates a relatively homogeneous grouping of discharges. Notwithstanding the need to analyze the MDC 15 relative weights further, there is a sufficient pattern of substantial differences in the relative weights to warrant further investigation of the implications of using the HCFA relative weights to allocate IME funds.

REGRESSION ANALYSES

Table 8 provides an overview of the regressions that we include in this report and identifies the table in which the results are reported for the first time. (We repeat the results of some regressions in several tables to facilitate comparisons with other regression results.)

Fully Specified Regressions

We report the results for selected fully specified regressions in Table 9. Model A and Model B compare the results using total cost per case as the dependent variable. Both regressions include the HCFA CMI and residents-to-average daily census as the teaching measure.

- As expected, the discharge-weighted regression (Model A) has a higher r-square than the facility-weighted regression (Model B).
- In both models, the case mix index, the wage index, percentage of outlier days, and the percentage of admissions through the emergency room are positive and highly significant.
- The CMI coefficients are greater than an expected value of 1.0, which indicates that the HCFA CMI is compressed. The compression means that the CMI overstates the costs of lower weighted DRGs and

understates the costs of higher weighted DRGs. Since teaching
hospitals tend to have higher than average case mix indices, the
compression creates an upward bias in the teaching coefficient.

- The wage index value, particularly in Model B, is considerably
  less than its expected value of 1.0 based on .72 labor-related
  share. It means that the wage index overstates the resources
  required by hospitals in higher-wage areas.

Table 9: Fully Specified Regression Results Using Average Cost Per Discharge for All Discharges as Dependent Variable Comparing Weighted Regression Using HCFA CMI and R2ADC as Measure of Teaching Intensity With Regressions Substituting No Weighting, R2Beds, or Pediatric CMIs

Variable	Model A Discharge-weighted HCFA CMIs Residents-to-ADC		Model B Facility-weighted HCFA CMIs Residents-to-ADC		Model C Discharge-weighted HCFA CMIs Residents-to-Beds		Model D Discharge-weighted Pediatric CMIs Residents-to-ADC	
	Coeff	T-stat	Coeff	T-stat	Coeff	T-stat	Coeff	T-stat
HCFA CMI	**1.233**	27.409	**1.184**	27.566	**1.229**	27.422	**1.252**	38.278
Wage index	**.786**	8.088	**.498**	4.386	**0.754**	7.718	**.942**	11.302
Teaching	**.210**	3.522	**.519**	8.422	**0.322**	4.15	**.171**	3.355
Low-income	**.265**	3.144	.148	1.546	**0.267**	3.195	**.175**	2.423
ADC	.023	1.503	**-.052**	-4.342	0.018	1.164	-.013	-1.001
Rural	**.096**	2.444	.051	1.557	**0.089**	2.244	.064	1.907
Large urban	**-.068**	-2.862	-.010	-.365	**-0.067**	-2.844	.009	.439
Proprietary	**-.090**	-2.875	**-.085**	-2.893	**-0.091**	-2.923	**-.118**	-4.408
Trauma center	**.005**	2.81	**.059**	2.444	0.004	0.194	-.014	-.773
FTEs/AdjADC	**.163**	5.418	**.068**	3.217	**0.159**	5.336	**.114**	4.436
% outlier	**4.524**	15.507	**3.429**	11.701	**4.524**	15.691	**2.639**	10.067
% ER admissions	**.768**	7.433	**.773**	11.256	**0.742**	7.147	**.263**	2.891
Intercept	**6.994**	72.567	**7.508**	104.321	**7.026**	72.192	**7.168**	88.292
r-square	.7900		.6720		.7909		.8461	

In Model A, all remaining explanatory variables other than hospital
capacity (ADC) are also significant. Hospitals located in large urban
areas are about 6.5 percent less costly than other hospitals and rural
hospitals are about 10 percent more costly than other hospitals. This
contrasts with Model B. When the regression is not weighted, the

coefficient for ADC is significant and negative and the coefficients for large urban, rural and serving low-income patients are not significant.

In both models, the coefficient for residents-to-average daily census is significant and positive. However, the coefficient is larger and more significant in Model B. Cost per discharge increases 2.1 percent for each .10 increment in the resident-to-bed ratio in Model A. It increases 5.2 percent for each .10 increment in the resident-to-bed ratio in Model B where there is no weighting. We obtain similar results using other measures of teaching intensity. To illustrate, we substitute residents-to-beds for residents-to-average daily census in a discharge-weighted regression in Model C.

- The r-squares for Models A and Model C are similar.
- The coefficient for residents-to-beds is slightly more significant. A hospital's cost per discharge increases 3.2 percent for each .10 increment in the resident-to-bed ratio. The higher coefficient in Model C relative to Model A reflects that each hospital's resident-to-bed ratio is lower than its resident-to-average daily census ratio.

Given the similarity of results, we report other fully specified regression results using the resident-to-average daily census teaching intensity measure only.

Model D substitutes the Pediatric CMI for the HCFA CMI in a discharge-weighted regression.

- The r-square increases from .790 (Model A) to .846.
- The CMI coefficient is similar to Model A's but is more significant.
- The wage index coefficient increases to .942 (std. error = .08) and is no longer statistically distinguishable from 1.0.
- The coefficient for teaching decreases from .21 to .17.
- Consistent with the increase in the significance of the CMI, other explanatory variables that also serve as a proxy for patient severity that is not explained by the case mix classification system are less significant (low-income, % outlier days, % emergency room admissions) or no longer significant (trauma center)

- The negative coefficient for proprietary hospitals increases in size and significance.

Variable	Model A All cases		All cases other than MDC 15		MDC 15 cases only	
	Coeff	T-stat	Coeff	T-stat	Coeff	T-stat
HCFA CMI	**1.233**	27.409	**1.275**	24.567	**1.072**	22.125
Wage Index	**0.786**	8.088	**0.589**	7.064	**0.918**	6.825
Res-to-ADC	**0.210**	3.522	**0.332**	6.872	-.008	-0.085
LIP	**0.265**	3.144	**0.402**	5.267	0.115	0.979
ADC	0.023	1.503	**0.031**	2.507	**0.057**	2.606
Rural	0.096	2.444	0.038	1.194	0.046	0.815
Large urban	**-0.068**	-2.862	0.024	1.140	**-0.099**	-3.002
Proprietary	**-0.09**	-2.875	-0.036	-1.251	**-0.188**	-4.453
Trauma	**0.005**	2.81	-0.014	-0.809	0.020	0.694
FTEs/ADC	**0.163**	5.418	**0.022**	4.007	**0.047**	5.296
% outlier	**4.524**	15.507	0.097	.464	**8.562**	22.199
% ER admissions	**0.768**	7.433	**0.295**	3.868	**0.166**	1.028
Intercept	**6.994**	72.567	**7.737**	101.684	**6.357**	51.214
r-square	0.7900		0.7035		0.7680	

Table 10: Fully-specified Regression Results Comparing All Discharges, All Discharges Other Than MDC 15, and MDC 15 Discharges Only As Dependent Variable Using HCFA CMI and R2ADC With Other Explanatory Variables

Given our concerns with MDC 15, we also perform separate fully specified regressions for other than MDC 15 discharges and MDC 15 discharges only. We compare the results of discharge-weighted regressions for these subsets of discharges with Model A in Table 10. The facility-level variables are identical to those used in Model A.

- The r-squares are lower in the separate regressions than in Model A when all discharges are included.
- The r-square for the regression using MDC 15 only discharges is higher than the r-square for the regressions that exclude MDC 15 discharges.

- The CMI coefficient for non-MDC 15 discharges remains compressed while the CMI coefficient for MDC 15 discharges is closer to its expected value of 1.0.

- The size and significance of the coefficients for teaching and outliers are quite different in the two regressions. For MDC 15 discharges only, the outlier percentage is highly significant while teaching is not. For all other discharges, teaching is significant while the outlier percentage is not.

- The MDC 15 results are dominated by the high volume of DRG 391 cases as well as extremely costly "outlier" newborns in other MDC 15 DRGs.

PAYER REGRESSIONS

In the payer regressions, we retain the following explanatory variables: case mix index, wage index, teaching, outlier percentage, and the proportion of low-income patients. We retain these variables because they are consistently significant in the fully specified discharge-weighted regressions and have been used by either MedPAC or the Medicare program in regressions to estimate the IME factor.

We perform a series of regressions examining the effect of using different measures of teaching intensity and adding additional explanatory variables. We include only the HCFA CMI, WI, and TI as explanatory variables in the models reported in Table 11. Model 1 uses ln (1+residents-to-average daily census) as the measure of teaching intensity. Relative to the Model A fully specified regression:

- The r-square decreases from .790 to .733 with fewer explanatory variables.

- The wage index coefficient is not statistically distinguishable from its expected value of 1.

- The CMI coefficient is 1.6 compared to an expected value of 1.0. The increase in the size and significance of the CMI coefficient reflects the dropping of other explanatory variables that are a proxy for patient severity.

- For the same reason, there is an increase in the size and significance of TI. The TI coefficient increases from .21 in Model A to .747 in Model 1.

What is the effect of using a different measure of teaching intensity?

	Table 11: Payer Regression Results Comparing Alternative Teaching Measures With HCFA CMI and WI Without Controlling for Outliers Using Cost Per Discharge for All Discharges As Dependent Variable							
Variable	Model 1 Residents-to-ADC		Model 2 Residents-to-Beds		Model 3 Residents-to-Adjusted ADC		Model 4 No. Residents	
	Coeff	T-stat	Coeff	T-stat	Coeff	T-stat	Coeff	T-stat
HCFA CMI	**1.604**	38.09	**1.598**	38.11	**1.613**	38.02	**1.569**	38.15
Wage index	**.905**	10.21	**.859**	9.487	**.919**	10.18	**.895**	10.37
Teaching	**.747**	13.36	**.988**	13.70	**1.008**	12.82	**.082**	15.28
Intercept	**7.903**	356.9	**7.909**	364.13	**7.914**	360.0	**7.836**	330.3
r-square	. 7328		.7344		.7209		.7423	

Table 11 compares the results of regressions using different measures of teaching intensity along with the HCFA CMI and WI as explanatory variables. The form of the teaching variables is ln (1+ratio). As previously noted, Model 1 uses residents-to-average daily census as the TI measure. Model 2 uses ln (1+ residents-to-beds ratio). Well newborn nursery beds are included in the bed count consistent with the HRSA policy for counting these beds. The Model 2 results are similar to those for Model 1. [14]

- The r-squares are very slightly higher in the Model 2 regressions.
- The TI coefficient is .988 when residents-to-beds is used in Model 2 compared to .747 in Model 1 when residents-to-average daily census is used. The difference is consistent with the

---

[14] We also evaluated the effects of using the Medicare definition of residents-to-beds that excludes well newborn nursery bassinets in the denominator to see whether the definitional difference affects the results. We found a slight reduction in the TI coefficient, which is expected since the ratio of residents-to-beds is higher without well newborn bassinets in the denominator. The r-square is also slightly lower; therefore, we use only the HRSA definition (which includes well newborn bassinets in the denominator) in subsequent regressions.

resident-to-bed ratio being lower than the resident-to-average daily census ratio.

In Model 3, the teaching intensity measure is residents-to-adjusted average daily census.

- With the inclusion of the adjusted discharges in the denominator of the TI measure, the coefficient is lower relative to using residents-to-ADC (Model 1).

- The r-square is also slightly lower than the other models.

In Model 4, we investigate using a teaching measure based solely on the number of residents (ln (1+no.of residents)). This definition appears to perform as well as the other measures of teaching intensity.

- The r-square is slightly higher than the r-squares for the other models.

- Teaching is slightly more significant than in the other models.

The similarity of the regression results across the alternative teaching measures suggest that the simulation results and policy considerations should determine which measure would be more preferable as the basis for an IME allocation factor. As discussed in the next section, we use the results from these regressions in our simulations of potential IME allocation factors for the CHGME program.

What is the effect of including additional explanatory variables?

Table 12: Payer Regression Results Using R2ADC As TI Measure With HCFA CMI and WI Comparing the Effect of Including Outlier or Low-Income Variable As Explanatory Variable

Variable	Model 1 Residents-to-ADC Only		Model 5 Residents-to-ADC With Outlier %		Model 6 Residents-to-ADC With Low-income	
	Coeff	T-stat	Coeff	T-stat	Coeff	T-stat
HCFA CMI	**1.604**	38.088	**1.330**	236.040	**7.860**	291.091
Wage Index	**.905**	10.211	**.644**	7.869	**.850**	9.295
Res-to-ADC	**.747**	13.364	**.413**	7.586	**.704**	12.379
Low Income	---	---	---	---	**.273**	3.049
% Outlier	---	---	**4.563**	16.869	----	---
Intercept	**7.903**	356.859	**7.489**	236.040	**7.860**	291.091
r-square	.7328		.7802		.7335	

We report in Table 12 the results of adding additional explanatory variables using residents-to-average daily census as our TI measure. We include the Model 1 results to facilitate the comparisons. Model 5 adds an outlier measure as an explanatory variable. The model is similar to MedPAC's except that the MedPAC model uses residents-to-beds as the TI measure. The outlier variable increases the r-square and makes a substantial reduction in the TI coefficient.

- The r-square is only slightly lower than in the fully-specified regression (.780 compared to .790).
- The TI coefficient is less significant and decreases from .747 to .413.

Model 6 drops the outlier variable and adds a measure for serving low-income patients. This model is similar to the one used by the Medicare program to estimate the IME adjustment for capital PPS except that the Medicare regression used a non-logged form of the teaching and low-income patient variables.

- Adding the low-income variable does not improve the r-square (.734) compared to Model 1 (.733).
- The size and significance of TI is slightly smaller in Model 6 relative to Model 1.

We use the payer regressions to estimate the IME effect on pediatric costs per discharge after controlling for factors that payers might be expected to take into account in paying for inpatient care. The most likely factors other payers are likely to take into account are the CMI and the WI. It is also highly likely that a payer is willing to pay more for outlier discharges, i.e., discharges with an atypical length of stay. For this reason, and because the outlier variable has a considerable effect on the r-square, we include the outlier variable in our remaining regressions. It is less likely that payers would take a hospital's service to low-income patients into account in determining payment amounts. Since the low-income patient variable does not improve the explanatory power of the regression (as measured by the r-square) and is not as likely to be recognized by other payers in paying for pediatric care, we drop the variable from the remaining payer regressions.

Using outliers as an explanatory variable has a similar effect of increasing the r-square and reducing the TI coefficient when other measures are used for TI (see Appendix Table A12).

What is the effect of using different forms of the TI measure?

Table 13 summarizes the results of regressions exploring different transformations of the TI measure. Model 5 is the regression that uses ln (1+residents-to-average daily census ratio) as the TI measure and includes the outlier percentage as an explanatory variable. Model 5A uses the form ln (.0001+ratio) as a means of reducing the bias in the coefficients. Model 5B uses the non-logged form of the measure. The r-squares are similar for all three measures and there are only slight variations in the coefficients for other than the teaching measure. The Model 5A coefficients are lower than the Model 5 coefficients because the scales are different.

Table 13: Payer Regression Results Comparing Effect of Different Forms of R2ADC With HCFA CMI, WI and Outliers Using Cost Per Discharge of All Discharges as Dependent Variable

Variable	Model 5 Residents -to- ADC ln(1+ratio)		Model 5A Residents -to- ADC ln(.0001+ratio)		Model 5B Residents-to- ADC non-logged	
	Coeff	T-stat	Coeff	T-stat	Coeff	T-stat
HCFA CMI	1.330	32.031	1.382	34.197	1.347	241.89
Wage index	.644	7.869	.729	8.994	.667	8.128
Teaching	.413	7.586	.018	5.937	.251	6.842
Outlier%	4.563	16.869	4.665	16.887	4.236	17.427
Intercept	7.489	236.04	7.650	198.78	7.514	241.89
r-square	.7802		.7766		.7780	

Figure 1 compares IME factors resulting from the regression coefficients for resident-to-average daily census ratios ranging from .05 through 1.50. (The range of ratios for children's teaching hospitals in our analysis file is from .05 to 1.54.)

- The IME factors derived from Model 5 ln (1+ratio) and Model 5B (non-logged) are fairly similar. Model 5 provides somewhat higher IME factors.
- The IME factors derived from Model 5A are much flatter.

Figure 1
Comparison of IME Specification Forms

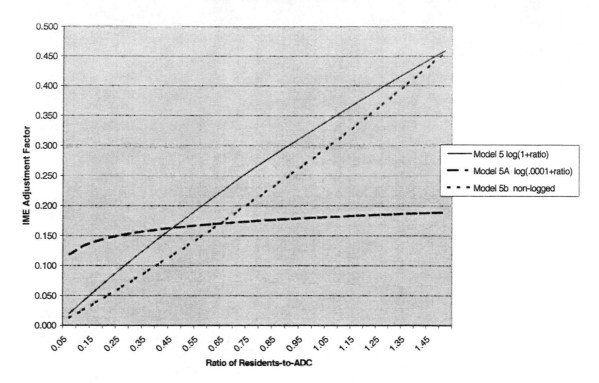

Model 5A would give considerably more weight to CMI and WI differences and little weight to increases in the teaching intensity ratio above .25 if it were used to allocate IME funds. The differences would affect individual hospital shares of the IME fund. Since Model 5 has a slightly higher r-square than the other two models, we use this form in our remaining regressions.

How Are Results Affected by Choice of Dependent Variable and CMI?

In Table 14, we compare regression results from Model 5 with models defining the dependent variables as the natural log of cost per discharge for 1) other than MDC 15 and 2) MDC 15 only discharges. In the results reported in Columns 3 and 4, the HCFA CMI is used. In the models reported in Columns 5 and 6, the Pediatric CMI is used.

- As was the case with the fully specified regressions, the r-squares are lower when the MDC 15 cases are treated separately.

- When the Pediatric CMIs are substituted for the HCFA CMIs, there is an increase in the r-squares. Other changes in the coefficients are in the expected directions. The CMI and wage index coefficients move closer to their expected values of 1.0 and the teaching coefficient is smaller.

- For MDC 15 discharges, the Pediatric CMI also reduces the size and significance of the outlier coefficient. In contrast, the outlier coefficient in the regressions for all discharges other than MDC 15 is higher using the Pediatric CMI than the HCFA CMI.

Table 14: Payer Regression Results Comparing All Discharges, Non-MDC 15, and MDC 15 Discharges As Dependent Variable With HCFA CMI or Pediatric CMI, WI and R2ADC As Explanatory Variables

(1) Variable	(2) Model 5 R2ADC All Discharges HCFA CMI		(3) R2ADC Non-MDC 15 Discharges HCFA CMI		(4) R2ADC MDC 15 Discharges HCFA CMI		(5) R2ADC Non-MDC 15 Discharges Pediatric CMI		(6) R2ADC MDC 15 Discharges Pediatric CMI	
	Coeff	T-stat	Coeff	T-stat	Coeff	T-stat	Coeff	T-stat	Coeff	T-stat
CMI	1.330	32.031	1.299	29.929	1.118	24.560	1.165	32.306	1.119	32.711
WI	0.644	7.869	0.713	10.812	0.680	5.891	0.802	12.467	.816	7.965
TI	0.413	7.586	0.489	12.056	0.246	3.083	0.439	11.078	0.179	2.544
Outlier%	4.563	16.869	.0355	1.833	8.852	24.956	0.530	2.867	5.727	16.433
Intercept	7.489	236.04	8.136	369.52	6.823	169.95	7.467	463.59	7.021	189.68
r-square	0.7802		.7169		0.7533		.7346		.8068	

ALLOCATION SIMULATIONS

We use the regression coefficients from the payer regressions to develop potential IME weighting factors for the CHGME fund. As discussed above in the Methods and Data section, the allocation weighting factor for each children's teaching hospital equal to:

$$WF_i = CMI_i^{\beta cmi} * WI_i^{\beta wi} * (TI_i^{\beta ti} - 1) * (NOD_i \text{ or } NOAD_i)$$

Each hospital's share of the IME fund equals its weighting factor as a percentage of the total weighting factors for all children's teaching hospitals:

$$\%IME_i = WF_i / \{ WF_i + WF_{ii} + WF_{iii} , , , $$

We limit our simulations to Models 1-4 reported in Table 11. We do not have the information needed to determine the outlier percentage needed to simulate models using outliers as an explanatory variable. The formulae that we use to develop the allocation weighting factors from Table 11 are:

Model 1: $WF_i = CMI^{1.604} * [(1+ R2ADC)^{.747} -1] *WI^{.905} * NOD$

Model 2: $WF_i = CMI^{1.598} * [(1+ R2Beds)^{.988} -1] *WI^{.859} * NOD$

Model 3: $WF_i = CMI^{1.613} * [(1+ R2AdjADC)^{1.008} -1] *WI^{.919} * NOAD$

Model 4: $WF_i = CMI^{1.569} * [(1 + FTE\ residents)^{0.082} -1] *WI^{.895} * NOAD$

For comparative purposes, we also simulate allocations based on the current payment adjustment factors used by the Medicare program for PPS operating payments and for PPS capital payments. We use the resulting allocation weighting factor from the PPS operating formula as our base model since it is the model that HRSA currently uses to allocate IME funds. The Medicare operating formula is similar to the formulae used to derive the allocation weighting factors from the regressions except it assumes that the wage index and CMI coefficients are equal to 1.0, the labor-related share is based on operating costs, and a multiplier is applied to the IME factor.[15] The formula is consistent with the way the payment adjustments are applied by the Medicare program. The formula is as follows:

$$WF_i = CMI_i * (WI_i * .711 + .289) * 1.6[(1+\text{residents-to-bed ratio}_i)^{.405} - 1] * NOD_i$$

The formula for determining a potential allocation weighting factor based on the Medicare capital adjustment factors is consistent with how the original regression equation was specified in developing the factors and the way the factors are applied by the Medicare program. The CMI coefficient is assumed to be 1.0, and the WI and TI factors are not logged. The formula for determining the weighting factor is:

$$WF_i = CMI_i * WI_i^{.6848} * (e^{.2822*\text{ratio of residents-to-ADC}} - 1) * NOD_i$$

---

[15] The IME factor is the difference between the amount a teaching and non-teaching hospital would receive holding all other factors constant. We account for this in the IME factor by subtracting 1 from the transformation of the regression coefficient, e.g., $1.0^{.405} = 1$.

We perform a total of six simulations and summarize the resulting distribution of IME funds by children's teaching hospital characteristics in Table 15. The current Medicare operating formula favors larger hospitals and hospitals with a large number of residents and/or high teaching intensity.

- Hospitals with an average daily census of 200 or more patients account for 15% of the discharges from children's teaching hospitals and receive 26% of the IME funds using this formula.

- Those with at least 100 residents account for 47.5% of pediatric discharges from children's teaching hospitals and receive slightly more than two-thirds of the IME funds under the Medicare operating formula.

The difference between the Operating and Capital Models reflects not only the change in the teaching intensity measure, but also a reduction in the relative importance of teaching (with the elimination of the multiplier) and a different methodology for applying the WI. When these changes are taken together, the Capital Model allocates additional funds to the larger hospitals and the larger residency programs. We would expect to see a reduction in the share of funds received by the hospitals with high occupancy rates because of the change from a resident-to-bed ratio to resident-to-average daily census ratio. However, this effect is not evident because of the other changes occurring simultaneously with the change in the teaching intensity measure.

Table 15 summarizes the net change in the distribution of IME funds across hospital classes. It does not provide information on the magnitude of the change for individual hospitals. To provide this information, we summarize in Table 16 changes in the share of the IME funds each hospital would receive relative to the Operating Model. For example, if the Capital Model were used to allocate funds:

- The share of the funds received by two hospitals would decrease between .25-.50 percentage points. The average decrease for the two hospitals is -.29 percentage points.

- Two hospitals would gain at least 1.0 percentage points. The average gain in their share of the IME funds is 1.47 percentage points.

Assuming 2/3 of the FY2001 appropriation is allocated for IME funds, each percentage point is about $1.56 million.

Across the remaining models, funds are redistributed among the classes of children's teaching hospitals as one would expect as the allocation formula changes. Table 15 shows the net changes within the various hospital classes are relatively small in moving from the Operating Model to Model 2, which reduces IME to an empirically justified level using the same teaching intensity measure (residents-to-beds). The biggest changes in the percentage of IME funds received by hospitals in a given category are for:

- the largest hospitals (28.2% vs. 26.3% under the Operating Model),
- hospitals with the highest case mix (28.5% vs. 26.7%), and
- hospitals with at least 100 residents (70.1% vs. 67.7 % in the Operating Model).

As seen in Table 16, each hospital's share of the IME fund would change by less than 1 percentage point.

In moving from an allocation based on residents-to-beds to one based on residents-to-average daily census (Model 1), the share of the IME funds received by low occupancy hospitals increases and the share of IME funds received by high occupancy hospitals decreases. Relative to the Operating Model, 27 hospitals would receive a higher share of the fund and 28 would receive a lower share. Each hospital's share would change by less than 1 percentage point.

- The share of the IME fund received by the 23 hospitals with an occupancy rate greater than 70 percent would decrease from 57.7 % to 53.0 % if Model 1 were used instead of the Operating Model.
- The share received by the 10 hospitals with an occupancy rate of less than 50 percent would increase from 5.8 % to 7.6 %.
- On average, smaller hospitals and those with smaller residency training programs receive a higher share of the IME

Table 15: Simulation of Distribution of IME Funds Using Regression Coefficients As Payment Parameters Compared to Using Medicare Formula

	Number of Hospitals	Number of Discharges	Estimated Share of IME Fund Allocation (%)					
			Medicare Operating Model	Medicare Capital Model	Model 1	Model 2	Model 3	Model 4
Average Daily Census								
LT 100	18	58,432	10.1	9.7	11.4	9.4	11.5	9.1
100-199	33	314,989	63.5	61.6	63.4	62.5	63.3	68.6
GE 200	4	67,014	26.3	23.7	25.2	28.2	25.2	22.3
Case Mix Index								
LT 1.15	8	56,965	8.6	8.1	8.7	7.3	8.7	9.8
1.15-1.19	13	102,488	19.8	19.6	19.8	18.7	19.9	20.1
1.20-1.29	21	164,373	44.9	46.8	43.1	45.4	43.1	38.8
GE 1.30	13	116,609	26.7	25.6	28.4	28.5	28.3	31.3
Number of Residents								
LT 10	11	32,962	0.7	0.6	0.8	0.6	0.7	2.6
10-99	27	198,306	31.6	28.8	33.2	29.3	32.8	38.5
GE 100	17	209,167	67.7	70.6	66.0	70.1	66.5	58.9
Resident-to-ADC Ratio								
LT .20	9	37,026	0.8	0.7	0.7	0.7	0.7	3.1
.20-.49	16	120,827	16.8	14.9	15.7	15.8	15.1	24.9
.50-.74	13	121,855	25.7	24.0	26.7	25.4	25.0	30.1
GE .75	17	160,727	56.6	60.5	56.9	58.1	59.2	42.0
Occupancy Rate								
LT .50	10	37,347	5.8	5.5	7.6	5.1	7.7	5.9
.50-.69	22	186,450	36.5	35.3	39.4	36.2	39.5	41.2
GE .70	23	216,638	57.7	59.2	53.0	58.7	51.3	52.9
Medicaid Utilization								
LT .20	10	108,589	24.4	23.3	25.5	25.0	25.5	27.0
.20-.39	15	91,042	15.4	14.5	15.5	14.0	15.5	16.0
GE .40	14	89,135	16.7	16.2	16.8	16.7	16.7	19.9
Missing	16	151,669	43.6	46.0	42.2	44.3	42.3	37.1

Table 16: Summary of Hospital Gains and Losses of IME Funds Using Regression Coefficients To Establish Allocation Factors Relative to Using Medicare Formula For Operating Costs

Percentage Point Difference From Allocation Using Medicare Formula	Capital Model			Model 1			Model 2		
	N Hospitals	Discharges	Mean Percentage Point Difference	N Hospitals	Discharges	Mean Percentage Point Difference	N Hospitals	Discharges	Mean Percentage Point Difference
Hospitals Receiving Less Funds									
1.00 or more									
.50 to 1.00	2	29,646	-0.29	3	47,168	-0.68			
.25 to .50				6	60,050	-0.34	1	10,311	-0.43
0 to .25	44	193,532	-0.11	19	151,386	-0.12	40	289,996	-0.10
Hospitals Receiving More Funds									
0 to .25	5	10,101	0.10	18	98,986	0.09	8	63,342	0.08
.25 to .50	1	8,943	0.30	6	55,051	0.36	4	47,997	0.36
.50 to 1.00	1	12,496	0.54	3	27,794	0.72	2	28,279	0.70
1.0 or more	2	17,434	1.47						

Percentage Point Difference From Allocation Using Medicare Formula	Model 3			Model 4		
	N Hospitals	Discharges	Mean Percentage Point Difference	N Hospitals	Discharges	Mean Percentage Point Difference
Hospitals Receiving Less Funds						
1.00 or more	2	31,186	-1.30	3	49,490	-2.93
.50 to 1.00	2	27,608	-0.80	6	55,729	-0.86
.25 to .50	5	48,424	-0.37	3	25,655	-0.32
0 to .25	21	154,508	-0.09	10	69,687	-0.09
Hospitals Receiving More Funds						
0 to .25	15	78,430	0.09	13	48,452	0.06
.25 to .50	6	64,343	0.32	10	79,201	0.39
.50 to 1.00	4	35,936	0.76	5	64,874	1.50
1.0 or more						

- fund under Model 1 than under the Operating Model and Model
  2.

Across the classes of children's teaching hospitals, there is
little change in the proportion of funds received by each hospital class
between Model 1, which is based on residents-to-average daily census,
and Model 3, which is based on residents-to-adjusted average daily
census.

- The share of the IME fund received by the 17 hospitals with a
  resident-to-average daily census ratio of .75 or higher would
  increase from 56.9% under Model 1 to 59.2 % under Model 3.

- Two hospitals' share of the fund would be reduced by an
  average 1.77 percentage points and two others would have a
  loss of more than .50 percentage point relative to the
  Operating Model.

- The share received by four hospitals would increase an
  average of .76 percentage points.

The potential redistributions of IME funds are the greatest under
Model 4, which uses the number of residents as the teaching measure and
adjusted discharges as the volume measure.

- The percentage of the fund received by six hospitals would
  decrease on average by 2.93 percentage points; the percentage
  received by another 6 hospitals would decrease between .5 and
  1.0 percentage points.

- The share received by 15 hospitals would increase by .5
  percentage points or more.

- The share of the IME fund received by hospitals with the
  highest resident-to-average daily census ratio drops from
  56.6% in the Operating Model to 42.0 %.

- The fund share of the nine hospitals with the lowest
  resident-to-average daily census ratio of increases from 0.8
  % in the Operating Model to 3.1%.

- The formula also shifts funds to hospitals with small
  residency programs. The share received by the hospitals with
  at least 100 residents decreases from 67.7 % to 58.9% while

the share received by hospitals with fewer than 10 residents increases from 0.7 % in the Operating Model to 2.6 %.

- Hospitals with an average daily census of 200 or more patients receive 26.3% of the IME funds under the Operating Model. This share drops to 22.3 %.

IME COST ESTIMATE

Our reference model for estimating total IME costs is the IME costs derived from the Medicare payment methodology; that is, we first estimate what the IME adjustment would have been if the children's teaching hospitals had been paid under the Medicare prospective payment system in 1997 using the current Medicare formula[16]. To do so, we use the Medicare standardized amounts for capital and operating costs and apply the payment adjustment factors applicable to each hospital. Next, we estimate total IME costs for each children's teaching hospital using the coefficients from our regression results. We use the same regression models and coefficients that we use in our simulation models. Except for the addition of the intercept coefficient, the formula for each model is identical to that used to establish the weighting factors. (The intercept was unnecessary in determining the weighting factors since it is a constant.) For example, the formula for Model 1 is:

$$\text{IME Cost}_i = e^{7.903} * \text{CMI}^{1.604} * ((1 + \text{R2ADC})^{.747} - 1) * \text{WI}^{.905} * \text{NOD}$$

Our results are summarized in Table 17. The average wage and CMI-adjusted cost per discharge represents the average cost per discharge for a non-teaching hospital located in the same geographic areas as children's teaching hospitals and with the same case mix. The average IME adjustment factor is the discharge-weighted average IME factor for children's hospitals derived from the regression. These factors are all considerably higher than the Medicare factor. Even though they are applied to a lower average wage and CMI-adjusted cost per discharge, the discharge-weighted average additional cost is higher. The per discharge additional cost ranges from $1,650 in Model 4 to $2,774 in Model 3

---

[16] Since the 1997 calendar year overlaps two fiscal years, we use a weighted average of the FY1997 (.75) and FY1998 (.25) standardized amounts for operating and capital costs applicable to the hospital's location in a large urban or other area.

compared to $1,393 in the Medicare Model. The estimates using residents-to-average daily census (Model 1) and residents-to-beds (Model 2) are about $830 million. The aggregate IME estimates are higher when adjusted discharges are used as the measure of hospital capacity. These estimates are based on an assumption that teaching has the same impact on outpatient services as inpatient services. While this is an empirical question, our ability to analyze it is hampered by the lack of case mix information for outpatient services. If only inpatient discharges were used in the estimate, the total amounts would be about 1/3 lower. (Inpatient discharges are about 2/3 of adjusted discharges.)

The IME estimate does not indicate the funding needed to "level the playing field" for children's teaching hospitals. However, it can provide information on the percentage of IME costs that are subsidized by the CHGME fund. Assuming $156 million (2/3 of $235 million) of the CHGME funds are allocated for IME funding, the funding level would have covered about 19 percent of inpatient IME costs using Models 1 or Model 2 and about 25% of IME costs using the Medicare model. The estimates are based on the regression models that include only teaching along with the HCFA CMI and WI as explanatory variables and would be lower if outliers or a more refined case mix classification were used.

Table 17: Estimates of IME Costs of Children's Teaching Hospitals In 1997 Based on Regression Coefficients for Selected Regression Models Compared to Current Medicare Formula

Model	Average WI+CMI-Adjusted Cost Per Discharge	Average IME Adjustment Factor	Average IME Adjustment Per Discharge	Total Estimated IME Costs
Medicare	$5,562	25.0 %	$1,393	$620 M
Model 1	$4,004	47.9%	$1,877	$830 M
Model 2	$4,016	46.3%	$1,862	$827 M
Model 3	$4,047	68.6%	$2,774	$1,231M
Model 4	$3,698	43.0%	$1,590	$1,066M

4. DISCUSSION OF MAJOR FINDINGS

MAJOR FINDINGS

This report uses multivariate regression analysis to investigate the effect of residency training programs on pediatric costs per discharge using different measures of teaching intensity. The study uses the coefficients from payer regressions to establish potential IME allocation formulae that could be used by the CHGME program and to estimate the aggregate IME costs of children's teaching hospital. Key findings include the following:

- In fully specified regressions that include a full set of explanatory variables, the teaching variable is a significant factor in explaining differences in costs per discharge for pediatric patients. In discharge-weighted regressions, cost per discharge increases 2.1 percent for each .10 increment in the ratio of residents-to-average daily census.

- The inclusion or exclusion of other explanatory variables has a significant effect on the size of the teaching coefficient. In particular, the variable for outlier cases (defined as atypical cases with long lengths of stay) has a strong influence on the teaching coefficient. When outlier cases are included in a payer regression, cost per case increases 4.13 percent for each .10 increment in the residents-to-average daily census ratio. When outlier cases are excluded, cost per case increases 7.47 percent for each .10 increment in the ratio.

- The regression results indicate that improvements in the case mix index would improve the teaching estimates. When the pediatric CMI is substituted for the HCFA CMI in the fully specified regressions, the significance of CMI increases while the coefficients for both the teaching and outlier variables decrease significantly.

- The choices between using residents-to-beds or residents-to-average daily census as the measure of teaching intensity and between using different forms of these measures (e.g., logged or non-logged) do not produce marked differences in the size of the teaching estimate. The teaching effect on cost per discharge is lower when the number of residents is used as the teaching measure and higher when the ratio of residents-to-average daily census is adjusted for outpatient volume.

- The choice of teaching measure affects the distribution of IME funds across children's teaching hospitals. Using the Medicare formula as the baseline, the largest redistribution occurs when the allocations are based on the number of residents only.

- The estimate of total IME costs at children's teaching hospitals for inpatient services only is dependent on the other factors included in the estimate. For inpatient services only, total IME costs are an estimated $830 million using either residents-to-average daily census or residents-to-beds as the teaching measure and controlling for case mix and geographic wage differences only. This compares to $620 million using the Medicare payment parameters.

DISCUSSION AND CONCLUSIONS

From a policy perspective, the most important issue is what methodology should be used to allocate IME funds across children's teaching hospitals. We believe the study results indicate that the Medicare IME formula is a reasonable basis for allocating IME funds under the CHGME program. For the most part, the allocations are similar to those based on pediatric costs per case using either residents-to-beds or residents-to-average daily census as the teaching measure. Nevertheless, there are aspects of the methodology that warrant further investigation. In particular, refinements in case mix measurement could improve the estimates of IME costs and how the IME funds are allocated across children's teaching hospitals.

Several areas of inquiry in this report were limited by the lack of patient-level data for children's teaching hospitals. The HCUP KID database became available as this study was nearing completion and could be used to answer several questions raised by the study.

- Additional work is needed to understand the differences in the HCFA relative weights and those derived from the pediatric cost data. Having children's hospitals represented in the database would enrich the analysis. Differences in cost structures could be accounted for by using the hospital-specific relative value method to establish the relative weights.

- The dominant effect of the MDC 15 DRGs (and DRG 391 in particular) on the regression results warrants further investigation since children's teaching hospitals have relatively fewer discharges assigned to MDC 15. The HCUP KID database could provide hospital-level information on the distribution of HCFA DRGs for this analysis.

- The regression results indicate using relative weights specific to pediatric discharges improves the IME estimate. However, we did not have the data to determine if using the Pediatric CMIs would result in a significant reallocation of IME funds across children's teaching hospitals. The HCUP KID data could be used to analyze this issue as well as the issue of whether more refined DRGs (e.g., TRICARE/CHAMPUS or APR-DRGs) would affect the allocation.

- The regressions results were also sensitive to the inclusion or exclusion of an outlier variable. Again, the HCUP KID data could also be used to examine the issue of how including an outlier variable would affect the allocations to children's teaching hospitals. It could also be used to examine the impact of including other variables, such as the low-income patient variable, in the allocation methodology.

Another area that warrants additional attention concerns outpatient services. The simulation results indicate that switching to a teaching measure that takes outpatient volume into account could involve significant reallocations for some children's teaching hospitals. The adjustment that we investigated for outpatient volume assumes the IME effect on outpatient services is comparable to the effect on inpatient services. This is an empirical question that would benefit from further analysis. However, the lack of consistent measures of outpatient volume and case mix will make it difficult to explore this issue in the near future.

APPENDIX A

Table A12: Payer Regression Results Comparing Alternative Measures of Teaching Variable With HCFA CMI, WI and Outliers Using Cost Per Discharge for All Discharges As Dependent Variable								
Variable	Residents-to-ADC		HRSA Residents-to-Beds		Residents-to-Adjusted ADC		No. Residents	
	Coeff	Coeff	Coeff	T-stat	Coeff	T-stat	Coeff	T-stat
HCFA CMI	**1.330**	32.031	**1.315**	31.735	**1.339**	31.943	**1.343**	32.958
Wage index	**.644**	7.869	**.598**	7.264	**.670**	8.031	**.672**	8.300
Teaching	**.413**	7.586	**.585**	8.418	**.563**	3.522	**.043**	7.800
Outlier%	**4.563**	16.869	**4.545**	17.038	**4.524**	15.507	**4.304**	15.216
Intercept	**7.489**	236.04	**7.487**	237.21	**6.994**	72.567	**7.487**	236.17
r-square	.7802		.7823		.7697		.7807	

REFERENCES

Anderson GF. Lave J. R. "Financing Graduate Medical Education Using Multiple Regression to Set Payment Rates," *Inquiry*, 23 (1986): 191-99

Averill R, et al., "The Evolution of Casemix Measurement Using Diagnosis Related Groups (DRGs)" in Norbert Goldfield, M.D., Editor, <u>Physician Profiling and Risk Adjustment</u>, 2nd Edition, Aspen Publishers, 1999.

Commonwealth Fund Task Force on Academic Health Centers. "Leveling the Playing Field: Financing the Mission of Academic Health Centers." The Commonwealth Fund, 1997.

Council on Graduate Medical Education. "Fifteenth Report:Financing Graduate Medical Education in a Changing Healthcare Environment," Rockville, Maryland: U.S. Department of Health and Human Services, 2000.

Dalton K., Norton E. C. "Revisiting Rogowski and Newhouse on the Indirect Costs of Teaching: A note on functional form and retransformation in Medicare's payment formulas," *Journal of Health Economics*, 2000a.19 (16): 1027-46

Dalton,K., E.C. Norton, and K. Kilpatrick, "A Longitudinal Study of the Effects of Graduate Medical Education on Hospital Operating Costs," *Health Services Research*, 2000b; 35(6):1267-1291).

Department of Health and Human Services, Health Care Financing Administration.

"FY 1992 Annual Update to the Medicare PPS Rates," Federal Register, 1991:56(169): 43380.

Department of Health and Human Services, Health Care Financing Administration. "Medicare Program: Prospective payment system for hospital outpatient services: Proposed rules," Federal Register, 1998: 63(173): 47581.

Department of Health and Human Services, Health Resources and Services Administration, HHS. "Children's Hospitals Graduate Medical Education (CHGME) Program," Federal Register, 2000a; 66(41): 12940.

Department of Health and Human Services, Health Resource and Services Administration. "Children's Hospitals Graduate Medical Education (CHGME) Payment Program: Final Methodology for Determination of FTE Resident Count, Treatment of New Children's Teaching Hospitals, and Calculation of Indirect Medical Education Payment," Federal Register, 2001b; 66(140):37980.

Goldfarb MG, Coffey RM. Case-Mix Differences Between Teaching and Nonteaching Hospitals, Inquiry, 24 (Spring 1987): 68-84.

Mechanic R., Coleman K, and Dobson A. Teaching Hospital Costs Implications for Academic Missions in a Competitive Market, JAMA, vol. 280, no. 11, September 1998.

Medicare Payment Advisory Commission. "Report to the Congress: Selected Medicare Issues." Washington, D.C.: MedPAC, June 2000.

Muldoon JH. Structure and Performance of Different DRG Classification Systems for Neonatal Medicine, Supplement of Evidence-Based Quality Improvement in Neonatal and Perinatal Medicine, Pediatrics, 103(1) January 1, 1999.

NACHRI, "Summary of Current Status of All-Patient Refined-Diagnosis Related Groups (APR-DRGS)," September 21, 1999.

Rogowski JA and Newhouse JP. "Estimating the indirect costs of teaching," Journal of Health Economics, 11 (1992): 153-173.

Personal communication . Craig Lisk, MedPAC staff..

Phillips SM. "Measuring teaching intensity with the resident-to-average daily census", Health Care Financing Review, vol. 14, no, 2, Winter 1992.

Sheingold SH. "Alternatives for using multivariate regression to adjust prospective payment rates," *Health Care Financing Review*, vol.11, no. 3, Spring 1990.

Thorpe KE. "The use of Regression Analysis to Determine Hospital Payment: The Case of Medicare's Indirect Teaching Adjustment," *Inquiry*, 25 (summer 1988): 219-231

Welch W P." Do all Teaching Hospitals Deserve an Add-On Payment under the Prospective Payment System?," *Inquiry*, 24 (Fall 1987): 221-232.

Zwanziger J, Sloss EM, Hosek SD, Bamezai A, Davis LM, Cameron KM, Prospective Payment for CHAMPUS Exempt Services:An Analysis of Children's Hospitals, Substance Abuse Services, and Psychiatric Services," RAND/WD-4096-1-HA, 1992.